FRCA: passing the primary examination

D1337889

FRCA: passing the primary examination

Dr Hugh Williams, registrar, MBBS
Dr Maan Hasan, consultant, MBChB, FRCA
Dr Michael Brunner, consultant, MBBS, FRCA
Dr Neville Robinson, consultant, MBChB, FRCA

Department of Anaesthesia, Northwick Park and
St Mark's Hospitals, Harrow, Middlesex HA1 3UJ

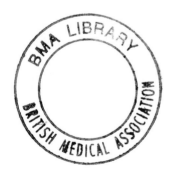

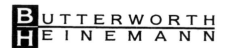

BUTTERWORTH
HEINEMANN

Butterworth-Heinemann
Linacre House, Jordan Hill, Oxford OX2 8DP
A division of Reed Educational and Professional Publishing Ltd

Ɛ A member of the Reed Elsevier plc group

OXFORD   BOSTON   JOHANNESBURG
MELBOURNE   NEW DELHI   SINGAPORE

First published 1996

© Reed Educational and Professional Publishing Ltd 1996

British Library Cataloguing in Publication Data
A catalogue record for this book is available from
the British Library.

Library of Congress Cataloguing in Publication Data
A catalogue record for this book is available from
the Library of Congress.

ISBN 0 7506 3108 2

Typeset by BC Typesetting, Bristol BS15 5YD
Printed and bound in Great Britain by
Biddles Ltd, Guildford and King's Lynn

Contents

Introduction

Why are you looking at all the MCQ books in this bookshop?

We think we know the answer and can help you because we were in the same situation not too long ago. Have you done enough study? What's the exact standard of the exam? Have you covered the syllabus? Will the examiners be fair? Can you cope with the stress of the vivas? Will Arsenal win the league? All are reasonable questions and your anxiety will be increased by stories of misery and horror that senior anaesthetists will tell you about 'the exam in their day'.

This is not just another MCQ book!!! The object of this companion text is to help you pass the exam. It is filled with sensible advice about the syllabus, the MCQs, the vivas and the OSCEs. Practice exams are included with relevant advice about how to pass this professional exam.

The exam is expensive (about £250) and ideally, you've invested about 18 months of your life preparing for it. Failure is a miserable experience. This book is set to the examination standard and will help give you confidence and understanding of what's required of you.

Good luck!!!

The exam

As from 1 August 1996 the Fellowship of the Royal College of Anaesthetists (FRCA) became a two-part exam. The first part is the Primary and the second part is the Final. There are two sittings per year for each part of the exam.

Are you eligible to sit for the Primary FRCA?

You need to satisfy four requirements:
- Be registered (full or temporarily) with the GMC.
- Be registered with the College as a post-graduate trainee in anaesthesia.
- Have 1 year's approved training in anaesthesia in the UK or Irish Republic.
- Satisfy the appropriate requirements of the application procedure (this essentially means filling out the application form correctly and writing a hefty cheque).

(If you are not eligible to sit the old Part 1 exam you are not eligible to sit the Primary FRCA.)

How do you apply?

The Royal College of Anaesthetists will send you, free of charge, an examinations calendar. Write to the Examinations Department, Royal College of Anaesthetists, 48–49 Russell Square, London WC1B 4JY.

Apply on time. The fee to sit the exam is expensive. You should not spend it just having a go. There is no point in sitting and failing the exam several times, as the only benefit to you personally will be a set of very expensive HB pencils that you will have done the MCQs with. They ask you to leave the rubber behind but the pencil is a legacy! Make sure when you apply that you write your cheque to the Royal College of Anaesthetists and sign it. You can also send a sterling draft, postal order or eurocheque.

What happens if you withdraw?

Should you feel this desire before the closing date, write to the examinations department and your money will be refunded. The College will deduct some administration expenses. If you withdraw under any other circumstances or fail to appear you will not normally be reimbursed. In exceptional circumstances (such as being on a ventilator, meningitis!) your request may be met by a sympathetic response.

How is the exam marked?

For each part of the exam you will be given 1 of 5 marks. The system used is

2+	good pass
2	pass
1+	fail
1	poor fail
0	veto

The following marks are required to pass the exam: 2, 2, 2, 1+ or better. A mark of 1 or less is an automatic fail. If you acquire this sort of mark in the MCQs and thereby make it impossible to pass the exam as a whole, you will not be allowed to attempt the vivas or OSCEs (you will receive no refund – the College cellars need constant restocking!).

The examiners do not know how you have got on in the other parts of the exam when you are sitting the vivas and OSCEs. They have not seen your marks. Candidates seem notoriously bad at marking themselves. Often after failing the exam a candidate will express the view that they were terrible in viva 1 but good in viva 2, only to find that the examiners marked it the other way around. The message is 'do not mark yourself and do not fail yourself.'

What is the structure of the exam?

The exam is in four parts.

1. 90 MCQs of 3 h duration consisting of:

- 30 questions in pharmacology.
- 30 questions in physiology and biochemistry.
- 15 questions in physics and clinical measurement.
- 10 questions in clinical anaesthesia.
- 5 questions in statistics.

2. Objectively Structured Clinical Examination (OSCE) with 16 stations in 2 h consisting of stations in:

- Resuscitation.
- Technical skills.
- Procedural anatomy.
- Regional anaesthetic block anatomy.
- History taking.
- Physical examination.
- Communication.
- Interpretation of results of tests.
- Anaesthetic equipment.
- Monitoring devices.
- Measuring equipment.
- Anaesthetic hazards.

3. Viva 1, of 30 min duration consisting of:

- 15 min in pharmacology and statistics.
- 15 min in physiology and biochemistry.

4. Viva 2, of 30 min duration consisting of:

- 15 min in physics, safety, clinical measurement.
- 15 min in clinical topics, e.g. critical incidents.

What happens if you fail?

Ideally don't. Should the cruel hand of fate descend upon you then sit the exam again. The examiners send you a run-down of your performance. You can sit the exam a maximum of four times. After two failures you cannot sit for a third time without guidance. With the candidate's consent, two things happen. Firstly, the College will receive a confidential report by your College Tutor and secondly, you will have to attend guidance sessions arranged by the College.

You can appeal (prior to the next closing date of the exam) if you feel you have been maltreated by the system. Write to the Examinations Director (not an individual examiner) about your problem.

Don't cheat. It leads to expulsion and if found out at a later date, will lead to the withdrawal of your diploma.

The syllabus

After a minimum of 12, but ideally 18 months in a recognized training post, a trainee may attempt the exam. General knowledge of the whole syllabus is desirable. Detailed knowledge in a few areas to the exclusion of good, basic knowledge is obviously silly. The syllabus can be divided into nine sections.

1. Equipment.
2. Clinical anaesthesia:
   - regional
   - general
3. Resuscitation and trauma.
4. Anatomy.
5. Physiology.
6. Pharmacology.
7. Physics.
8. Clinical measurement.
9. Statistics.

The Royal College of Anaesthetists has given guidelines about the syllabus. Your senior colleagues will tell you endlessly how lucky you are to have a syllabus, as in their day there was no syllabus, no textbooks, and the exam was much more difficult, with a 15% pass rate etc. This will tend to wear you out, but bear with it as you will probably do the same when you become a consultant.

1. Equipment

All of the pieces of equipment that you use every day in anaesthesia or intensive care are basic to the speciality and you must know them. Everything in anaesthesia is designed for a purpose and you must develop the capacity to think and ask 'why?' as you proceed in the subject. For example, why is the laryngoscope designed as it is? The light, blade, and handle can all be shaped and positioned differently.

You will be required to understand the following:

- Principles of anaesthetic machine function.
- Checking the anaesthetic machine.
- Cylinders.
- Manufacture of gases.
- Pipelines.
- Suction devices.
- Scavenging systems.
- Anaesthetic breathing systems.
- Electrical safety.
- Monitoring devices.
- Minimal monitoring standards.
- Tracheal tubes.
- Laryngeal masks.
- Airways.
- Oxygen masks.
- Cannulae.
- Transfusion devices.
- Principles of pulmonary ventilators.

You will fail if fundamental subjects such as checking the anaesthetic machine are not word perfect – start with the oxygen analyser and how it works.

The most difficult subject in this section is 'transfusion devices' which will lead into a discussion of blood transfusion including its indications and complications.

2. Clinical anaesthesia

Clinical anaesthesia is a huge topic and for the sake of ease regional anaesthesia will be dealt with first. Remember, all anaesthetics can be done either using general and/or regional anaesthesia.

Regional anaesthesia

- Spinal anaesthesia.
- Epidural anaesthesia.
- Caudal anaesthesia.
- Intravenous regional anaesthesia.
- Brachial plexus block.
- Femoral nerve block.

- Ilio-inguinal nerve block.
- Local anaesthesia for tracheal intubation.

A helpful way of approaching this subject is to consider the anatomy, the indications, the contraindications, resuscitation equipment, place to perform block, drugs to be used with toxicity, actual technique, effects, and complications. Common side effects should be mentioned first. As regards epidurals, for example, the easiest way of discussing the complications is to mention hypotension first, then accidental intravenous injection, followed by dural puncture – not massive spinal, infection etc. Clarity of thought helps here and you should have performed all of the above blocks. (See viva section for further information about this topic.)

General anaesthesia

As with all general anaesthetics, this subject can be divided into its components for ease of learning.

Preoperative assessment

- Drug therapy and its implications (e.g. beta blockers, MAOIs).
- Drug allergies and their implications.
- Personal and family history of anaesthetic problems and its implications.
- Problems in emergency anaesthesia assessment.
- Assessment of the airway and degree of difficulty of tracheal intubation.
- Assessment of hydration.
- Guidelines for restriction of smoking, food, and fluids.
- ASA classification.
- Glasgow coma scale assessment.
- Other pre-anaesthetic scoring systems.
- Interpretation of preoperative investigations – haematology, biochemistry, blood gases, ECGs, x-rays, pulmonary function tests.
- Problems of assessing and performing anaesthesia in medical diseases, especially cardiac (valvular disease, myocardial infarction, and angina), respiratory (asthma and chronic bronchitis), vascular (hypertension), blood diseases (sickle cell and anaemia), renal disease, and endocrine diseases (diabetes mellitus).
- Electrolyte disorders.

- Problems of anaesthesia in surgical diseases (intestinal obstruction, trauma and the acute abdomen).
- Assessment and management of acute trauma.

Premedication

- Indications for premedication.
- Choice of drugs and their advantages and disadvantages.

Induction

- Techniques of induction – inhalational versus intravenous, advantages and disadvantages.
- Indications for intubation.
- Management of failed intubation.
- Management of difficult intubation.
- How to manage potentially difficult intubations.
- Tracheal intubation – correct tracheal tube placement, oesophageal intubation, endobronchial intubation.
- Regurgitation and vomiting.
- Cricoid pressure – indications and technique.
- Pulmonary aspiration.
- Post-intubation wheeze.
- Diagnosis and management of anaphylactoid and anaphylactic reactions.
- Induction in special circumstances – head injury, full stomach, and upper airway obstruction.

Intraoperative

This will include the ability of the anaesthetist to deal with anaesthetically and surgically induced emergencies before, during and after anaesthesia. How to stabilize a patient before senior assistance arrives will also be assessed.

- Techniques of maintenance – analgesia, prevention of awareness.
- Management of ventilation and relaxation.
- Intraoperative fluid therapy.
- Monitoring.
- Diagnosis and management of critical incidents especially:
  cyanosis
  hypertension
  hypotension
  cardiac arrhythmias

    bronchospasm
    respiratory obstruction
    increased peak inspiratory pressure
    pneumothorax
    hypercarbia
    hypocarbia – gas embolism, air embolism
    failed intubation
    failed reversal of relaxation

- Definition and management of massive haemorrhage.
- Hazards of blood transfusion.
- Malignant hyperthermia.
- Causes of failure to breathe at the end of operation.
- Suxamethonium apnoea.

Postoperative

- Management of the unconscious patient.
- Care in the recovery room.
- Complications after extubation especially:
      failure to awaken
      confusion
      stridor
      inadequate respiration
      shivering
      hypertension
      hypotension
- Oxygen therapy – indications and techniques.
- Postoperative fluids.
- Prevention, diagnosis and treatment of DVT and pulmonary embolus.
- Postoperative nausea.
- Postoperative analgesia methods and assessment.
- Vomiting.

Anaesthesia in special circumstances

- Principles of obstetrics.
- Children (not neonates) including ENT, eye and dental procedures.
- Day surgery.
- Management of head injuries.
- Obesity.
- Repetitive anaesthesia – hepatic injury.
- Implications of HIV and hepatitis.

3. Resuscitation and trauma

The guidelines of the Resuscitation Council will be followed and the immediate care and resuscitation of patients (all ages) is required.

- Patient assessment.
- Principles and practice of life support.
- Management of life-threatening arrhythmias (drug therapy and defibrillation).
- Venous and intra-osseous access and complications.
- Airway and ventilation.
- Paediatric resuscitation problems.
- Ethics in resuscitation.

In trauma, the management of hypovolaemic shock and its consequences will be examined.

- Pathophysiology.
- Assessment, immediate care, and management (all ages).
- Primary and secondary survey.
- Specific management of abdominal and thoracic trauma.
- Airway and oxygen therapy.
- Vascular access.
- CVP management.
- Pneumothorax and chest drain insertion.
- Analgesia for trauma patients.

4. Anatomy

Anatomy relevant to anaesthesia will be asked. This is occasionally absolutely factual but is more often applied to clinical practice. Learning anatomy by heart is often the only way in which to do it, but it should be considered as part of the whole subject. Learning, e.g. the anatomy of the inguinal canal, is more interesting if considered within the subject of anaesthesia for repair of inguinal hernia including regional techniques available.

Respiratory system

This is important and if you cannot describe the views seen at laryngoscopy you will fail.

- Mouth, nose, pharynx, *larynx, trachea*, main bronchi, segmental bronchi.
- Pleura, mediastinum.
- Lungs, lobes, *bronchopulmonary segments*.
- *Innervation of respiratory tract*, blood supply, lymph drainage.
- Muscles of respiration, *diaphragm*.

Cardiovascular

- Pericardium.
- *Heart – conducting system, blood supply*.
- *Fetal circulation*.
- Peripheral vessels.

Nervous system

- Brain and structure of the spinal cord.
- Meninges.
- *Cerebrospinal fluid*.
- *Epidural space*.
- *Subdural space*.
- Spinal nerves.
- Dermatomes.
- Cervical plexus.
- *Brachial plexus*.
- Nerves to the arm.
- *Intercostal nerves*.
- Lumbar plexus.
- *Nerves to the abdominal wall*.
- *Sacral plexus*.
- *Coccygeal plexus*.
- Nerves to leg.
- *Autonomic nervous system*.
- *Stellate ganglion*.
- *Coeliac plexus*.
- Cranial nerves.
- Trigeminal ganglion.

Vertebral column

- *Vertebrae*, especially the *lumbar*.
- *Sacrum*.
- Ligaments.

Special areas

- *Thoracic inlet.*
- *First rib.*
- Paravertebral space.
- *Intercostal space.*
- *Inguinal canal.*
- *Abdominal wall.*
- Veins (neck, arm, leg).
- Diaphragm.
- Axilla.
- *Eye* and *orbit.*
- *Tracheostomy.*

5. Physiology

It is suggested that good knowledge of theoretical and applied physiology, especially with regards to anaesthesia, exists. There are 13 systems of knowledge required.

General

- Cell function.
- Cell membrane.
- Organization of the body and its control.
- Ageing.

Haematology

- Red cells, white cells and platelets.
- Haemoglobin and its variants.
- Blood groups.
- Allergy.
- Immunity.
- Inflammation.
- Haemostasis.
- Coagulation.

Muscle

- Action potential.
- Skeletal muscle.
- Cardiac muscle.

- Smooth muscle.
- Neuromuscular junction.

Heart

- Regulation and rhythmicity.
- Electrocardiogram.
- Cardiac output.

Circulation

- Blood pressure control.
- Blood volume control.
- Blood flow and measurement.
- Vascular endothelium.
- Pulmonary circulation.
- Coronary circulation.
- Cerebral circulation.
- Visceral circulation.
- Fetal circulation.

Body fluids and constituents

- Capillaries.
- Interstitial fluid.
- Intracellular fluid.
- Extracellular fluid.
- Total body water.
- Osmolarity.
- Osmolality.
- Lymphatics.
- Cerebrospinal fluid.

Kidneys

- Glomerular function.
- Plasma clearance.
- Tubular function.
- Urine formation.
- Fluid and electrolyte balance.
- Acid – base balance.

Respiration

- Oxygen transport.
- Carbon dioxide transport.
- Gaseous exchange.
- Regulation of respiration.
- Mechanics of respiration.

Nervous system

- Nerves and synapses.
- Sensation.
- Pain pathways.
- Motor function.
- Brain stem.
- Cerebellum.
- Cortical functions.
- Limbic system.
- Reflexes.
- Special senses.

Gastrointestinal

- Gut motility and reflexes.
- Gastric function.
- Vomiting and nausea.
- Digestion.

Metabolism and temperature

- Carbohydrate, fat, and protein metabolism.
- Hormonal control.
- Liver function.
- Control of temperature.
- Obesity.
- Starvation.
- Vitamins.
- Minerals.

Endocrinology

- Pituitary.
- Thyroid.
- Adrenal glands.

- Pancreas.
- Parathyroid and calcium.

Pregnancy

- Normal pregnancy changes.
- Placental function.

6. Pharmacology

This includes general pharmacology, a knowledge of anaesthetic drugs, and an understanding of drugs that patients may be on when they present for anaesthesia. Basically, the subject is divided into two categories; general and systematic. Most of the vivas are taken up with general pharmacology – subjects like receptors, log dose response curves are much more likely than a discussion on thiopentone. You must know definitions.

Applied chemistry

- Types of intermolecular bonds.
- Diffusion laws.
- Solubility coefficients.
- Partition coefficients.
- Drug ionization.
- Isomers.
- Protein binding.

Mode of drug action

- Receptors: agonists, antagonists, receptor binding.
- Potency.
- Efficacy.
- Tolerance.
- Drug enzyme interactions.
- Michaelis–Menton equation.
- Types of ion channels.
- Gating mechanisms.
- Drug actions.
- Membranes: action of gases and vapours.
- Osmotic effects.
- pH effects.
- Absorption.

- Chelation.
- Oxidation.
- Reduction.
- Mechanisms of drug interactions.
- Enzyme induction and inhibition.
- Addition, subtraction and synergism.
- Effects of metabolites.

Pharmacokinetics

- Bioavailability.
- Drug uptake from the gastrointestinal tract.
- Drug uptake from skin.
- Drug uptake by tissues especially muscle, CSF, subcutaneous, epidural space.
- Distribution of drugs.
- Drug uptake by the lung.
- Influence of drug formulation on disposition.
- Body compartments.
- Drug disposition to organs and tissues – tissue binding and solubility.
- Distribution in CSF and extradural space.
- Maternal–fetal distribution.
- Modes of drug elimination – phase 1 and 2 excretion.
- Pharmacokinetic analysis:
  pharmacokinetic compartment
  apparent volume of distribution
  clearance
  Fick principle
  compartmental models
  perfusion and partition coefficients
  variation including body size, sex, age, disease, pregnancy, anaesthesia, trauma, surgery, alcohol, and other drugs
- Pharmacodynamics – concentration effect relationships.
- Hysteresis.
- Pharmacogenetics – familial variation in drug response.
- Adverse reactions – idiosyncracy, hypersensitivity, allergy, anaphylaxis, anaphylactoid reactions.

Systematic pharmacology

The following have to be learnt relatively completely. It is quite a good idea to have a logical sequence when learning drugs – the physical properties, followed by chemical properties, then the systems affected and finally metabolism. What are the ideal properties of an anaesthetic intravenous agent, an inhalational agent, a neuromuscular blocking agent and an analgesic? What is the difference between a sedative and a hypnotic?

- Anaesthetic gases.
- Anaesthetic vapours.
- Hypnotics.
- Sedatives.
- Intravenous anaesthetics.
- Opioids and other analgesics.
- Neuromuscular blocking drugs.
- Non-steroidal anti-inflammatory drugs.
- Autonomic nervous system drugs – cholinergic and adrenergic agonists and antagonists.
- Drugs acting on the heart.
- Antihypertensives.
- Anticonvulsants.
- Diuretics.
- Antibiotics.
- Corticosteroids and hormones.
- Antacids and drugs acting on gastric secretion and motility.
- Antiemetics.
- Local anaesthetics.
- Plasma volume expanders.
- Antihistamines.
- Antidepressants.

7. Physics

The physical principles upon which clinical measurement is based will be examined. These principles need to be considered in relation to appropriate clinical factors, e.g. exponential functions need to be considered as a whole as they are important in volatile agent wash-in–wash-out curves, temperature measurement, preoxygenation, some drug metabolism (half-lives), lung inflation, and bacterial growth. Mostly this section is basic and it is a shame when candidates get confused about derived units such as pressure. Pressure is a derived SI unit, force per unit area, and the SI unit is the pascal (not kilopascal – you need to know this when you check an anaesthetic machine). Learn the following.

- Mathematical concepts – sinusoids, exponentials, parabolas.
- Basic measurement – linearity, drift, hysteresis, signal:noise ratio, dynamic response.
- SI units – fundamental, derived.
- Simple mechanics – mass, force, work, power.
- Heat – conduction, convection, radiation.
- Physics of gases – pressure, gas laws, density, viscosity, laminar and turbulent flow.
- Bernoulli principle.
- Freezing point, melting point, latent heat.
- Vapour pressure.
- Basic electricity and magnetism.
- Capacitance, inductance, impedance.
- Amplification.
- Processing, storage of physiological measurements.
- Lasers.
- Pacemakers.
- Defibrillators.
- Electrical hazards – electrocution, fires, explosions.
- Diathermy safety standards (BS5724).
- Pressure transducers.

8. Clinical measurement

The items that are used in clinical practice daily will be examined, as well as those in the ITU setting. The most important aspect of this is getting the items in a logical order for discussion and description, e.g. there are indirect and direct ways of measuring pressure and the examiner will be looking for the limitations of each as well as a basic understanding of how the equipment works. Do not forget respiratory function tests. Remember that you must be able to define absolute and relative humidity – what is its relevance to anaesthesia? How can you humidify gases? The hardest part of this is the measurement of carbon dioxide and oxygen only because they appear as gases and in blood. Once this distinction is made, it becomes pretty clear and straightforward to learn.

- Measurement of pressure.
- Measurement of volume and flow in gases and liquids.
- Pneumotachograph.
- Peak flow measurement.
- Spirometry.

- Temperature.
- Humidity.
- Measurement of gas concentrations – oxygen, carbon dioxide, nitrogen, nitrous oxide, volatile anaesthetic agents.
- Measurement of pH, pCO_2, pO_2.
- Pulmonary function tests.
- Capnography.
- Pulse oximetry.
- Measurement of neuromuscular blockade.
- Assessment of pain.

9. Statistics

Do *not* omit this section. Occasionally candidates think that they will be able to pass without any understanding of this subject. There are five MCQs and almost certainly you will be asked about this in the vivas. Basic statistical knowledge is required. This is to ensure that you can understand research papers and assess them critically. In all likelihood, research will be carried out at some time in an anaesthetist's career (if you're really lucky!!). Understanding statistics then becomes fundamental.

Emphasis is placed on the methods used by which data is presented and which statistical measurements are used for different types of data. Knowledge of measurement errors and statistical uncertainty is required. One way of doing this is to read the journals and try to understand why certain statistical tests were chosen.

- Categories of data.
- Statistical distributions (gaussian, chi squared, binomial).
- Non-parametric measures of location and variability.
- Graphical representation of data.
- Simple probability theory.
- Confidence intervals.
- Linear correlation.
- The null hypothesis.
- Type one and two errors.
- Probability of error occurrence.
- Choice of tests for different data types.

You have now finished the syllabus! Go to the pub because you are no doubt suicidal!!!

3

The MCQs

The MCQs test your factual knowledge in more depth than the other parts of the exam. Apart from knowing the subject, all you can do to prepare is to do as many past papers and practice MCQs as you can get your hands on.

The exam will consist of 90 stem questions, each with five possible responses which will be true or false. You will have 3 hours to complete them. There will be 30 physiology and biochemistry, 30 pharmacology, 15 physics and clinical measurement, 10 clinical anaesthesia and 5 statistics questions.

When you start the exam, spend some time understanding how to fill in the computer answer form correctly (the rest is easy). Three hours is a long time, so you should easily finish all the questions. Don't rush. Take time reading the stem questions. It is easy to misinterpret the question and give the wrong answers to a question you may well know the answer to.

If you ask ten people about MCQ technique, you will probably get 15 answers. The only advice we can give is when you have answered all the questions that you can, *stop*, even if there is still time. Don't be tempted to guess as the questions are negatively marked. That means you lose points for a wrong answer. Having said that, an educated guess is more likely to be correct than incorrect. If any of the questions are ambiguous, don't be afraid to ask the examiner to clarify it for you.

The rest of this chapter contains 180 MCQ questions. The first 90 questions will be divided into sections to allow you to practise different topics separately:

30 pharmacology
30 physiology and biochemistry
15 physics and clinical measurement
10 clinical anaesthesia
 5 statistics.

The second 90 MCQs will contain a mix of questions as in the exam proper. You should not spend more than 3 hours on this.

Pharmacology (30)

1. Pulmonary vascular resistance (PVR) is reduced by:

A   Alpha sympathomimetic drugs.
B   Beta sympathomimetic drugs.
C   Aminophylline.
D   Sodium nitroprusside.
E   5-HT.

FTTTF
A,B,C,D,E PVR is increased by: hypoxia, hypercarbia, histamine, 5-HT and alpha sympathomimetics. It is reduced by isoprenaline, beta sympathomimetics, aminophylline and sodium nitroprusside.

2. Ketamine:

A   Anaesthetic dose is 1–2 mg/kg intravenously or 10 mg/kg intra-muscularly.
B   Is a potent analgesic.
C   Does not alter plasma catecholamine levels.
D   Does not alter the tone of skeletal muscles.
E   Is metabolized in the liver.

TTFFT
A   These are the commonly used doses for both children and adults.
B   Ketamine has profound analgesia (remember, thiopentone is not analgesic).
C   It commonly increases catecholamine levels, BP and heart rate.
D   It usually increases the tone of skeletal muscles.

3. The following are potassium sparing diuretics:

A   Frusemide.
B   Triamterene.
C   Amiloride.
D   Ethacrynic acid.
E   Spironolactone.

FTTFT
Potassium sparing diuretics are: triamterene, amiloride and spiro-nolactone.
A,D Hypokalaemia is a known side effect of these drugs. Both are potassium losing diuretics.

4. Thiopentone:

A   Is hypnotic but not analgesic.
B   Solution is acidic.
C   Is contraindicated in malignant hyperpyrexia.
D   Is contraindicated in porphyria.
E   Has an elimination half-life of about 30 min.

TFFTF

A   Sometimes even labelled as 'antanalgesic'.
B   Thiopentone is acidic but its solution is very alkaline (a pKa of 8 and a solution pH of 11).
C   Halothane and suxamethonium are among the contraindicated drugs in MH.
D   Elimination half-life is about 4–5 h (10–15% of the drug is metabolized each hour).

5. Cardioselective beta-adrenoceptor antagonists include:

A   Acebutalol.
B   Atenolol.
C   Propranolol.
D   Metoprolol.
E   Labetalol.

TTFTF

A,B,D   Cardioselective beta-adrenoceptor antagonists include: acebutalol, atenolol, metoprolol, practolol, and bisoprolol.
C   Propranolol is a beta 1 and 2, adrenoceptor antagonist.
E   Labetalol is a beta 1 and 2, and alpha adrenoceptor antagonist.

6. The following drugs have alpha adrenoceptor antagonist effects:

A   Prazocin.
B   Phenoxybenzamine.
C   Labetalol.
D   Sodium nitroprusside.
E   Phentolamine.

TTTFT

A,B,E   Phenoxybenzamine (long acting), phentolamine (short acting), prazocin, doxazocin, and terazocin are alpha adrenoceptor antagonists.

C Labetalol has both alpha and beta antagonism.
D Sodium nitroprusside is a direct vasodilator.

7. Alpha adrenoceptor agonism effects include:

A Bronchodilation.
B Increase in cardiac contractility.
C Increase in heart rate.
D Increase in arterial pressure.
E Stimulation of insulin secretion.

FFFTF
A,B These result from beta receptor agonism.
C,D Alpha agonism results in vasoconstriction, increase in systemic vascular resistance, increase in arterial pressure, and possibly reflex bradycardia.
E Alpha agonism causes inhibition of insulin secretion.

8. The following antihypertensive drugs have a central mechanism of action:

A Methyl dopa.
B Clonidine.
C Reserpine.
D Phenoxybenzamine.
E Minoxidil.

TTTFF
A,B,C Methyl dopa, clonidine and reserpine have significant central adrenergic-inhibitory effects. Clonidine and reserpine also have peripheral effects.
D This is an alpha adrenoceptor antagonist.
E This is a direct vasodilator.

9. Regarding antihypertensive drugs:

A Verapamil, nifedipine, nicardipine and diltiazem are all calcium channel entry blockers.
B Captopril, enalapril and minoxidil are all renin–angiotensin system inhibitors.
C Frusemide, bumetanide and ethacrynic acid are all loop diuretics.
D Amiloride, triamterene and spironolactone are all distal tubule diuretics.
E Trimetaphan, phentolamine and pentolinium are all ganglionic blockers.

TFTTF

B Minoxidil is a direct vasodilator. Captopril, enalapril, ramipril, cilazapril and lisinopril are renin–angiotensin system inhibitors.

D They are also potassium sparing diuretics.

E Phentolamine is an alpha adrenoceptor antagonist.

10. Volatile anaesthetics:

A Halothane and enflurane are halogenated hydrocarbons.

B Isoflurane has a higher boiling point than halothane.

C Halothane, isoflurane and enflurane are all metabolized to varying degrees.

D Enflurane is not used in epileptics.

E Enflurane is the agent of choice in patients with raised intracranial pressure.

FFTTF

Halothane is a halogenated hydrocarbon. Isoflurane and enflurane are halogenated ethers. The boiling point of enflurane is 56.5°C, isoflurane 48.5°C, halothane 50.5°C. The percentage metabolized is approximately 20% halothane, 2% enflurane, 0.2% isoflurane. Enflurane should be avoided in epileptics as hyperventilation with enflurane causes epileptiform activity on the EEG. Isoflurane is the agent of choice in raised intracranial pressure as it increases intracranial pressure to a lesser extent than halothane and enflurane.

11. The following agents are likely to be effective in reducing the tachycardia/hypertension response to laryngoscopy and intubation of the trachea:

A Propranolol.

B Sodium nitroprusside.

C Esmolol.

D Hydralazine.

E Labetalol.

TFTFT

A,C,E Beta adrenoceptor antagonists are known to be effective in reducing these responses to laryngoscopy and intubation.

B,D Nifedipine, sodium nitroprusside and hydralazine, like many other vasodilators, are not as effective in spite of their ability to control blood pressure prior to laryngoscopy and intubation.

12. Transfer of drugs across biological membranes is known to be influenced by:

A   Size of membrane pores.
B   Molecular weight of the drug.
C   Degree of ionization of the drug.
D   Drug–protein binding.
E   Concentration gradient of the drug across the membrane.

TTTTT
B   Molecular weights are usually used to determine the size of drug molecules.
C   The ionized form of the drug is water soluble and the union-ized form is lipid soluble. Remember, biological membranes are mainly lipid and the degree of drug ionization is dependent on its lipid/water solubility.
D   Normally only the free drug can cross biological membranes.

13. The following drugs undergo significant first pass effect:

A   Propranolol.
B   Atenolol.
C   Glyceryl trinitrate.
D   Lignocaine.
E   Pethidine.

TFTTT
Drugs that are extensively metabolized in the gut wall or the liver undergo first pass effect when given orally. The oral doses of such drugs are significantly higher than the injectable doses.
A   The oral dose of propranolol is significantly larger than the i.v. dose.
B   Atenolol is water soluble, does not undergo significant first pass effect and is excreted mostly unchanged in the urine.
C   Glyceryl trinitrate can be taken sublingually.
D   Lignocaine is extensively metabolized in the liver.

14. Regarding drug metabolism, the following are known to cause enzyme induction:

A   Phenytoin.
B   Barbiturates.
C   Benzodiazepines.
D   Chronic ingestion of alcohol.
E   Steroids.

TTFTT

A,B,D,E Drugs known to cause enzyme induction are: barbiturates (e.g. phenobarbitone), phenylbutazone, phenytoin, steroids and alcohol. Remember drugs known to cause enzyme inhibition are: MAO inhibitors, warfarin, chloramphenicol and alcohol.

15. The following are known allergenic agents:

A   Radiographic intravenous contrasts.
B   Dextrans.
C   Latex.
D   Althesin.
E   Etomidate.

TTTTF

C   Latex containing products have been blamed for contact dermatitis, allergic reactions and even anaphylactic reactions from direct IgE mediation.
D   Althesin and propanidid were withdrawn from anaesthetic practice because of high incidence of allergic reactions (approximately 1 in 10 000).
E   Amongst the commonly used intravenous anaesthetics and muscle relaxants, etomidate and vecuronium are probably the least likely to cause histamine release.

16. Regarding drug metabolism, the following are known to cause enzyme inhibition:

A   MAO inhibitors.
B   Alcohol.
C   Chloramphenicol.
D   Warfarin.
E   Phenytoin.

TTTTF

A,B,C,D Drugs known to cause enzyme inhibition are: MAO inhibitors, warfarin, chloramphenicol and alcohol.
E This causes enzyme induction rather than inhibition.

17. Drugs known to cause methaemoglobinemia include:

A   Nitrites.
B   Glutathione.
C   Prilocaine.

D Ascorbic acid.
E Sulphonamide compounds.

TFTFT
A,C,E Drugs known to cause methaemoglobinemia include: prilo-caine, nitrites, sulphonamides, methylene blue, phenacetin and acetalinide.
B,D These do the opposite (i.e. reverse methaemoglobinaemia). Methaemoglobinaemia is also reversed by the enzyme NADH methaemoglobin reductase (endogenous) and methylene blue.

18. Frusemide:

A Acts primarily by inhibiting sodium reabsorption in the proxi-mal tubule.
B Causes an increase in renal blood flow.
C Causes hyperkalaemia.
D Causes hypercalcaemia.
E Causes ototoxicity.

FTFFT
A Frusemide, a loop diuretic acts primarily by inhibiting the active reabsorption of sodium chloride in the thick ascending limb of the loop of Henle.
B Frusemide causes a prostaglandin mediated increase in renal blood flow.
C,D Increased loss of both potassium and calcium leads to both hypocalcaemia and hypokalaemia.
E Ototoxicity is a recognized complication.

19. The following drugs are more than 90% protein bound:

A Warfarin.
B Diazepam.
C Frusemide.
D Digoxin.
E Alcohol.

TTTFF
A,B,C Warfarin is more than 99% protein bound. Frusemide and diazepam are both 95–99% protein bound.
D,E Alcohol and digoxin are less than 50% protein bound.

20. Insulin:

A Is secreted by pancreatic alpha cells.
B The majority is secreted from the pancreas as preproinsulin.
C Raises intracellular potassium.
D Binds to nuclear receptors.
E Stimulates protein synthesis.

FFTFT
Insulin is secreted by pancreatic beta cells. It is initially synthesized as preproinsulin, a prohormone; however, before being released this is cleaved and the majority is released as insulin. Insulin causes potassium to enter cells. Insulin binds to a membrane bound insulin receptor. One of the recognized effects of insulin is increasing protein synthesis.

21. Features of non-specific drug receptors are:

A High capacity.
B Sensitivity.
C Saturability.
D Antagonism.
E High affinity.

TFFFF
A Non-specific receptors occupy large areas of cell membrane and have large capacity for drugs. They are also known to have low sensitivity and low affinity for drugs.
B,C,D,E These are features of specific drug receptors.

22. Doxapram:

A Acts upon peripheral chemoreceptors.
B Can cause a tachycardia.
C May be given as an infusion.
D Is useful in the treatment of status asthmaticus.
E Should be avoided in severe hypertension.

TTTFT
Doxapram is a respiratory stimulant which acts principally on the peripheral chemoreceptors, increasing their sensitivity to PaO_2. Administration can cause both hypertension and tachycardia. Doxapram may be given by both bolus and infusion. It is contra-indicated in status asthmaticus and severe hypertension.

23. Nitrous oxide:

A Has a molecular weight of 42.
B Is flammable.
C Is commercially produced by heating ammonium nitrate.
D Contamination by nitric oxide is detected by starch iodide paper.
E Has a critical temperature of −7°C.

FFTTF
A MW of $N_2O = 14 \times 2 + 16 = 44$.
B It is neither flammable nor explosive. However, it supports combustion of other agents even in the absence of oxygen because at temperatures >450°C it decomposes to nitrogen and oxygen.
E The critical temperature of nitrous oxide is 36.5°C; that of Entonox is −7°C.

24. Regarding antidiabetic therapy:

A A change of insulin, from an animal to human preparation, usually requires an increase in dosage of about 10%.
B A subcutaneous injection of soluble insulin produces peak effect in about 30 min.
C Soluble insulin has a half-life of about 5 min when injected intravenously.
D Compared to sulphonylureas, therapy with biguanides (metformin) is more likely to cause hypoglycaemic episodes.
E HbAlc of more than 7% is usually associated with good control.

FFTFF
A This may require a decrease rather than increase in the dose.
B This has an onset of effect in 20–30 min, peak effect in 2–3 h and duration of 4–8 h.
D On the contrary, due to its mechanism of action (stimulation of insulin secretion), sulphonylureas are more likely to cause hypoglycaemia. Metformin can cause lactic acidosis.
E This should read 'less than 7% is associated with good control'; normal HbAlc is 4–6%.

25. The following agents have cholinergic effects:

A Carbachol.
B Methacholine.

C   Edrophonium.
D   Pilocarpine.
E   Cyclopentolate.

TTTTF
A,B,C,D Cholinergic drugs include; acetylcholine, the synthetic choline esters (carbachol, bethanecol and methacholine), natural alkaloids (such as pilocarpine and muscarine), and anticholinesterases (such as edrophonium, physostigmine, neostigmine, pyridostigmine, ambenonium, and organo-phosphorous compounds.
E This is anticholinergic.

26. Concerning muscle relaxants, the following statements are true:

A   Rocuronium is a steroidal compound.
B   Mivacurium has a faster onset than rocuronium.
C   Mivacurium is not suitable for intravenous infusion.
D   Rocuronium is metabolized by pseudo-cholinesterase.
E   Vecuronium has significant vagolytic effects.

TFFFF
A   Steroidal compounds include; pancuronium, pipecuronium, vecuronium, and rocuronium.
B   Onset of rocuronium (60–90 s) is faster than that of mivacurium (2.5 min). Amongst non-depolarizing muscle relaxants, rocuronium is perhaps the closest to suxamethonium regarding rate of onset.
C,D Mivacurium is metabolized by plasma cholinesterase. It has a short duration of action. Repeated doses or infusion of mivacurium are not associated with delay in slope of recovery. Rocuronium is not metabolized to any significant extent. Instead, it undergoes dual renal and hepatic elimination.
E   Vecuronium is known for its cardiovascular stability. It has no vagolytic activity. However, such activity may be seen with other steroidal compounds such as pancuronium and to a lesser extent rocuronium.

27. The following are metabolized (partially or completely) by plasma cholinesterase:

A   Mivacurium.
B   Procaine.
C   Propandid.
D   Rocuronium.
E   Pipecuronium.

TTTFF
D,E Both rocuronium and pipecuronium undergo renal and hepatic elimination. They are not metabolized to any significant extent.

28. Aminoglycoside antibiotics:

A Cause defective protein synthesis in bacteria.
B Are bacteriostatic.
C Are active against anaerobes and aerobes.
D Do not cross the blood–brain barrier.
E Are poorly absorbed from the gut.

TFFTT
Aminoglycoside antibiotics bind to bacterial ribosomes causing defective protein synthesis, this effect is bactericidal. Aminoglycosides are ineffective against anaerobic bacteria. Aminoglycosides do not cross the blood–brain barrier and are poorly absorbed from the gut.

29. Etomidate:

A Is useful in patients with a limited cardiovascular reserve.
B Like methohexitone and propofol, produces pain on injection.
C Is commonly associated with allergic reactions.
D Produces excitatory movements.
E Is water soluble.

TTFTF
A Etomidate produces minimal cardiovascular depression and is therefore useful in patients with a limited cardiovascular reserve.
C Amongst intravenous anaesthetics it is probably the least allergenic.
B It produces pain on injection like methohexitone and propofol.
D Etomidate inductions are often associated with excitatory movements.
E Etomidate is presented in 35% propylene glycol as it is insoluble in water.

30. Penicillin G (benzyl penicillin):

A Is orally active.
B Intrathecal injection can cause convulsions.
C Is predominantly liver metabolized.

D May produce hypersensitivity reactions 2 weeks after administration.
E Is inactivated by beta lactamase.

FTFTT
A Benzyl penicillin is hydrolysed in the stomach.
B Very high intrathecal concentrations can cause convulsions.
C Benzyl penicillin is excreted by the kidney.
D Hypersensitivity reactions may be immediate or delayed, the
delayed reactions occurring within 1–2 weeks of treatment.
E One form of resistance to benzyl penicillin is inactivation by
beta lactamase.

Physiology and biochemistry (30)

1. The oxygen dissociation curve is shifted to the right by:

A An increase in temperature.
B Hypercarbia.
C An increase in 2,3-DPG enzyme.
D Metabolic alkalosis.
E Haemodilution.

TTTFF
A,B,C The oxygen dissociation curve is shifted to the right by:
increase in temperature, acidosis (metabolic or respiratory) and
increase in 2,3-DPG enzyme.
D Metabolic acidosis shifts the curve to the left.
E Haemodilution by itself has no effect on the affinity of Hb for
oxygen.

2. Pulmonary vascular resistance (PVR) is increased by:

A Hypoxia.
B Hypercarbia.
C Isoprenaline.
D Acetylcholine.
E Histamine.

TTFFT
A,B,C,D,E PVR is increased by: hypoxia, hypercarbia, histamine,
5-HT and alpha sympathomimetics. It is reduced by isoprenaline,
beta sympathomimetics, aminophylline and sodium nitroprusside.

3. Concerning the relationship between oxygen tension of the blood and oxygen saturation of haemoglobin, the following statements are true:

A   An oxygen tension of 110 mmHg or more is associated with 95–100% oxygen saturation of haemoglobin.

B   An oxygen tension of 60 mmHg is associated with 90% oxygen saturation of haemoglobin.

C   An oxygen tension of 40 mmHg is associated with 75% saturation of haemoglobin.

D   An oxygen tension of 20 mmHg is associated with 50% saturation of haemoglobin.

E   Respiratory or metabolic acidosis shift p50 to the left.

TTTFF

A,B,C,D,E Based on the oxygen dissociation curve; oxygen tensions (in mmHg) of 110 or more, 60, 40 and 27 (normally called p50) are associated with haemoglobin oxygen saturations of 95–100%, 90%, 75% and 50%, respectively. p50, like the rest of the curve, is shifted to the right by; an increase in temperature, acidosis and an increase in 2,3-DPG enzyme.

4. Regarding segmental cutaneous innervation of the body:

A   The umbilical area is supplied by T12.

B   The area of the xiphisternum is supplied by T3.

C   The inner aspect of the arm receives innervations from T1 and T2.

D   The hand receives innervations from C6, C7 and C8.

E   The anterior aspect of the upper thigh is mainly supplied by L2.

FFTTT

A   The umbilical area is supplied by T10.

B   The area of the xiphisternum is supplied by T6.

5. Cardiac output:

A   Is increased by acclimatization to high altitude.

B   Is increased by standing from the lying position.

C   Is increased in pregnancy.

D   Is reduced by i.v. infusion of sodium nitroprusside.

E   Is increased by i.v. infusion of isoprenaline.

TFTFT

A,B,C Cardiac output is increased by pregnancy and acclimatization to high altitude. Standing from the lying position reduces venous return and reduces cardiac output.

D,E Sodium nitroprusside increases cardiac output by reducing systemic vascular resistance (afterload). Isoprenaline increases cardiac output by increasing heart rate and contractility and also by reducing systemic vascular resistance (afterload).

6. Fibrinolysis is stimulated by:

A   Urokinase.
B   Aprotinin.
C   Tranexamic acid.
D   Streptokinase.
E   Alteplase.

TFFTT

A,B,C,D,E Fibrinolysis is stimulated by urokinase, streptokinase and alteplase. It is inhibited by antiplasmin, aprotinin, tranexamic acid or amino caproic acid.

7. Normal pregnancy at 32 weeks gestation:

A   Heart rate is increased.
B   Stroke volume is unchanged.
C   Diastolic arterial pressure is increased.
D   Central venous pressure is increased.
E   Plasma oncotic pressure is reduced.

TFFFT

A,B,C,D In normal pregnancy, cardiac output is increased, both heart rate and stroke volume are increased, and both peripheral vascular resistance and diastolic arterial pressure are reduced. Central venous pressure is usually unchanged.

E Plasma oncotic pressure is reduced mainly because of the reduction in plasma albumin.

8. In late pregnancy:

A   Respiratory rate is increased.
B   Tidal volume is decreased.
C   Airway resistance is not affected.
D   The functional residual capacity of the lungs is unchanged.
E   Arterial carbon dioxide tension is unchanged from the normal 5.3 kpa (40 mmHg).

TFFFF
A,B,C,D Both respiratory rate and tidal volume are increased.
Airway resistance is reduced, and the FRC is reduced.
E Arterial CO_2 tension is usually reduced by 5–10 mmHg.

9. The following are normal (not necessarily typical) physiological variables for a term newborn:

A Respiratory rate of 35 breaths/min.
B Tidal volume of 80 ml.
C Heart rate range of 80–110 beats/min.
D Blood volume of 300 ml.
E Haemoglobin of 18 g/dl.

TFFTT
A,B,C,D,E Normal physiological variables for a term newborn
are: respiratory rate of 25–40 breaths/min, tidal volume of 15–
25 ml, heart rate of 120–150 beats/min, blood volume of 300 ml,
and haemoglobin of 18 g/dl.

10. Concerning white blood corpuscles (WBC):

A Total count is $4–11 \times 10^9/l$.
B Differential count consists of 40–75% neutrophils.
C Differential count consists of 10–15% lymphocytes.
D Differential count consists of 5% basophils.
E Basophils contain granules of histamine and heparin.

TTFFT
A,B,C,D,E WBC total count is $4–11 \times 10^9/l$. Differential count is:
neutrophils 40–75%, lymphocytes 20–45%, monocytes 4–10%,
eosinophils 2–6%, and basophils less than 1%. Basophils contain
granules of histamine and heparin.

11. Daily requirements for a resting adult are:

A Carbohydrates 0.5 g/kg.
B Proteins 1 g/kg.
C Fat 0.5 g/kg.
D Sodium 1–2 mmol/kg.
E Potassium 1 mmol/kg.

FTFTT
A,B,C Daily requirement of proteins, carbohydrates and fats are 1,
2 and 2 g/kg, respectively.

D,E Daily requirement of sodium and potassium are 1–2 and 1 mmol/kg, respectively.

12. Regarding plasma proteins:

A Albumin, globulin and fibrinogen molecular weights are 69 000, 90 000–150 000, and 330 000, respectively.

B Plasma levels (g/l) of albumin, globulin and fibrinogen are 20–55, 15–30, and 10–15, respectively.

C Fibrinogen is the main contributor to plasma oncotic pressure.

D Globulin is the main contributor to plasma viscosity.

E Albumin is the main contributor (amongst plasma proteins) to erythrocyte sedimentation rate.

TFFFF

A Also, Hb (67 000) is slightly smaller than albumin; therefore in haemoglobinaemia it appears in urine.

B The range of albumin is 35–55 rather than 20–55 g/l, and fibrinogen is 2–4 rather than 10–15 g/l.

C Albumin is the main contributor to plasma oncotic pressure.

D Fibrinogen is the main contributor to plasma viscosity (remember the RBC is the main contributor to blood viscosity).

E Amongst the plasma proteins, fibrinogen is normally the main contributor to the ESR. However, in conditions of high plasma globulin, the latter may become more important.

13. The essential amino acids include:

A Leucine and isoleucine.

B Lysine and glycine.

C Tryptophan and trimethaphan.

D Methionine, threonine and phenylalanine.

E Histidine, valine and arginine.

TFFTT

The ten essential amino acids are: leucine, isoleucine, lysine, tryptophan, methionine, threonine, phenylalanine, histidine, valine and arginine.

B Glycine is not an essential amino acid.

C Trimethaphan is not an essential amino acid. It is a ganglionic blocker.

14. A 75 kg adult male at rest has approximately the following:

A Total body water of 45 l.

B Extracellular fluid of 15 l.
C Body surface area of 1 m^2.
D Cardiac index of 5 l/min per m^2.
E Energy requirement of 1200 kcal/day.

TTFFF
A Equivalent to 60% body weight.
B Equivalent to 20% body weight or one-third of total body water.
C About 2 m^2.
D About 3.2 l/min per m^2.
E About 2200 kcal/day (30 kcal/kg).

15. Breathing air at sea level; the following blood-gas values are typical or near typical:

A Mixed venous pCO$_2$ is 46 mmHg.
B Mixed venous pO$_2$ is 60 mmHg.
C Mixed venous O$_2$ saturation is 60%.
D Arterial bicarbonate is 26 mmol/l.
E Arterial total buffer base is 46 mmol/l.

TFFTT
A,B,C Typical mixed venous pCO$_2$, pO$_2$ and O$_2$ saturation are 46 mmHg, 40 mmHg and 75%, respectively.

16. Adrenaline:

A Is the transmitter at the sympathetic ganglia.
B Constitutes the main secretion from adrenergic neurones.
C Stimulates alpha, beta 1 and 2 adrenoceptors.
D Causes dilatation of the pupils.
E Is commonly used with local anaesthetics in a concentration of 1:20 000.

FFTTF
A Acetylcholine is the transmitter at sympathetic ganglia.
B Noradrenaline constitutes about 90% of the secretion from adrenergic neurones.
E This concentration with local anaesthetics is high. The correct concentration is 10 times weaker (i.e. 1:200 000).

17. The following are typical (or near typical) haemoglobin values:

A 18 g/dl for a newborn.

B 15 g/dl for a 6-month-old infant.
C 8.5 g/dl for a 1-year-old child.
D Less than 10 g/dl for an adult male known to have sickle cell disease.
E 14 g/dl for a term pregnant female.

TFFTF
A,B,C Normal values (g/dl) for haemoglobin are: 16–20 for newborn, 10–12 for a 6-month-old infant, 10.5–13 for a 1-year-old child, 12.5–17 for men, 11–15 for women, and 9.5–13.5 for pregnant women.
D Patients with sickle cell disease regularly suffer from haemolytic episodes. Their haemoglobin is usually found to be around 7–10 g/dl. Those with sickle cell trait usually have normal haemoglobin concentration.
E This is not typical. In pregnancy, the increase in blood volume exceeds the increase in the amount of haemoglobin resulting in low haemoglobin concentration. Haemoglobin range in term pregnancy is normally at 9.5–13 g/dl.

18. Examples of secondary messengers activated by drug-receptor interactions are:

A Cyclic adenosine monophosphate.
B Cyclic guanosine monophosphate.
C Calcium.
D Inositol.
E Calmodulin.

TTTTT
A,B,C,D,E Examples of secondary messengers are; CAMP, CGMP, calcium, inositol and calmodulin.

19. Insulin secretion is stimulated by:

A High blood sugar.
B Glucagon.
C Adrenaline.
D Neural sympathetic activity.
E Sulphonylureas and biguanides.

TTFFF
A,B Pancreatic beta-cell activity is stimulated by high blood sugar, glucagon or an increase in the neural parasympathetic activity.
C,D It is inhibited by adrenaline or neural sympathetic activity.

E Whilst stimulation of insulin secretion is the mechanism of action of sulphonylureas, metformin (the only available biguanide) works by decreasing gluconeogenesis and increasing peripheral utilization of glucose.

20. Regarding transport of oxygen in arterial blood:

A 1 g of saturated haemoglobin carries about 1.34 ml of oxygen.
B 100 ml of plasma carries about 0.3 ml of oxygen in solution (subject breathing air at sea level).
C 100 ml of plasma carries about 5 ml of oxygen in solution (subject breathing 100% oxygen at sea level).
D 100 ml of plasma carries about 20 ml of oxygen in solution (subject breathing 100% oxygen at 3 absolute atmospheric pressure).
E 100 ml of blood carries about 21 ml of oxygen (subject breathing 100% oxygen at sea level).

TTFFT
C,D 100 ml of plasma carries 1.8 and 6 ml of oxygen in solution when the subject is breathing 100% oxygen at sea level and at 3 absolute atmospheric pressure, respectively.

21. Concerning carbon dioxide:

A Alveolar tension is in equilibrium with mixed venous tension.
B In healthy adults, mixed venous tension is normally at 46 mmHg.
C 100 ml of arterial blood carries 24 ml of CO_2.
D For a given CO_2 tension, oxygenated blood carries more CO_2 than deoxygenated blood.
E CO_2 is carried in the blood in three different forms; simple solution, as bicarbonate, and as carbamino compound.

FTFFT
A Normally it is in equilibrium with pulmonary capillary tension or in near equilibrium with arterial tension (normally at 40 mmHg).
C It carries 48 ml of CO_2.
D Deoxygenated blood carries more CO_2 (Haldane effect) especially as carbamino compounds and bicarbonates.
E CO_2 is carried in the blood in three forms: in simple solution (constitutes about 5%), as bicarbonates (about 75%) and as carbamino compounds (about 20%).

22. Regarding transport of carbon dioxide in the blood:

A The enzyme carbonic anhydrase is abundant in both plasma and red blood cells.

B Carbonic anhydrase aids the combination of CO_2 and water to form carbonic acid.

C Carbonic anhydrase aids the breakdown of carbonic acid into CO_2 and water.

D A small proportion (about 5%) of CO_2 is carried as simple solution in plasma and the largest proportion of CO_2 is carried as bicarbonates.

E CO_2 combines protein molecules in the plasma and the red blood corpuscles to form carbamino compounds.

FTTTT

A The enzyme carbonic anhydrase is abundant in RBCs.

B,C Carbonic anhydrase speeds hydration of CO_2 into carbonic acid in the tissue side, and speeds the breakdown of carbonic acid into CO_2 and H_2O in the pulmonary side.

23. Transfer of a drug across the blood brain barrier is known to be influenced by:

A Its molecular weight.

B Its lipid solubility.

C Plasma drug–protein binding.

D Presence of a brain tumour.

E Encephalitis.

TTTTT

A Molecular weights usually determine the size of drug molecules.

B Remember biological membranes are mainly lipid. Drug ionization is also dependent on its lipid/water solubility.

C Normally only free drug can cross biological membranes.

D,E The blood–brain barrier can be distorted by a brain tumour or infection.

24. Prostaglandins:

A PGI_2 (prostacyclin) causes vasoconstriction and platelet aggregation.

B PGA_2 (thromboxane) causes vasodilation and platelet separation.

C PGF$_2$ causes bronchoconstriction and pulmonary vascular constriction.
D PGE$_2$ causes bronchodilation and pulmonary vascular dilation.
E PGE$_2$ and PGF$_2$ inhibit uterine action.

FFTTF
A Causes vasodilation and platelet separation.
B Causes vasoconstriction and platelet aggregation.
E They stimulate rather than inhibit the uterus.

25. The anterior pituitary gland secretes:

A Growth hormone.
B Oxytocin.
C Prolactin.
D Antidiuretic hormone (ADH).
E Adrenocorticotrophic hormone (ACTH).

TFTFT
A,C,E ACTH, TSH, FSH, LH, GH and prolactin are secreted from the anterior pituitary gland.
B,D Oxytocin and antidiuretic hormones are secreted from the posterior gland.

26. The adrenal cortex secretes:

A About 20 mg of cortisol per day (average adult).
B Testosterone.
C Androgen.
D Aldosterone.
E Spironolactone.

TFTTF
A,B,C,D The adrenal cortex secretes glucocorticoids (cortisol and corticosterone), mineralocorticoids (aldosterone) and sex hormones (mainly androgen).
E Spironolactone is a synthetic steroid diuretic. Remember it is a competetive antagonist of aldosterone.

27. Regarding the endocrine system, the following are true:

A Antidiuretic hormone (ADH) and oxytocin are secreted by the posterior pituitary gland.
B Thyroxine and calcitonin are secreted by the thyroid gland.

C Glucagon, insulin and somatostatin are secreted by the pancreas.
D Cortisol, aldosterone and androgen are secreted by the adrenal cortex.
E Renin, erythropoietin and 1,25-dihydroxycholecalciferol are secreted by the kidney.

TTTTT
B In addition, the thyroid gland secretes triiodothyronine.
D Also corticosterone.
E The kidney also secretes prostaglandins.

28. Antidiuretic hormone (ADH):

A Is a steroid hormone.
B Is also called vasopressin because of its pressor effects at high concentrations.
C Secretion is increased by a rise in osmolality of extracellular fluids.
D Secretion is increased by reduction in blood volume.
E Secretion is increased by morphine and decreased by alcohol.

FTTTT
A Is an octapeptide.
D This is controlled by stretch receptors in the atria and pulmonary veins.

29. Blood flow (as an approximate percentage of cardiac output) to organs of the body is as follows:

A 5% to the heart.
B 10% to the kidneys.
C 15% to the brain.
D 25% to the liver.
E 15% to fat tissues.

TFTTF
B Approximately 25% ($=1200$ ml/min).
E Fat has poor blood supply, approximately 5%.

30. Cerebrospinal fluid (CSF):

A Has a total volume of about 150 ml (average adult).
B Has a specific gravity of 1.005.
C Contains cells in a concentration of more than $5 \times 10^9/l$.

D Normally contains no proteins.
E Glucose level is usually lower than plasma glucose level.

TTFFT
A In an average adult, the CSF volume is about 150 ml, 50% of which surrounds the brain and the other 50% surrounds the spinal cord.
C Cells should be less than 5×10^9/l.
D Normal protein CSF level is 15–45 mg/100 ml.
E Glucose level is 2.5–4 mmol/l.

Physics and clinical measurement (15)

1. Regarding anaesthetic breathing systems:

A Lack and Bain systems are versions of Mapleson systems A and D, respectively.
B Fresh gas flow is delivered by the inner tube in both the Lack and Bain systems.
C The inner tube of the Lack system has a wider bore than that of the Bain system.
D The required fresh gas flow for the Bain system during spontaneous ventilation is approximately equivalent to 1 min ventilation.
E The only difference between Mapleson F and Mapleson E is the addition of an open-ended bag.

TFTFT
B,C The inner tube in the Bain system is narrow and delivers the fresh gas flow. The inner tube in the Lack system is the expiratory limb and therefore is made of a wider bore to reduce resistance to expiration.
D This is true for controlled ventilation. During spontaneous ventilation, a fresh gas flow of 2 × minute volume or more is required to prevent rebreathing.
E The Mapleson F is the Rees modification of the Mapleson E.

2. Concerning medical gas cylinders:

A A pressure reading of 133–140 × 100 kPa usually indicates a full O_2 cylinder.
B A pressure reading of about 50 × 100 kPa usually indicates a full N_2O cylinder.

C CO_2 filling pressure is about 50×100 kPa.
D Reducing valves are commonly used to reduce high cylinder pressure to 400 kPa.
E Gauge pressure equals absolute pressure.

TFTTF
A Full O_2 cylinder has a pressure of $133{-}140 \times 100$ kPa.
B N_2O filling pressure is about 50 atm. However, this reading does not necessarily indicate a full cylinder, as N_2O in the cylinder exists in both liquid and gaseous states. The pressure falls only when the cylinder is nearly empty. Weight of cylinder indicates degree of fullness.
C The same applies to CO_2.
E Cylinder gauges measure the relative pressure (above atmospheric pressure).

3. Soda lime:

A Contains approximately 94% calcium hydroxide, 5% sodium hydroxide, 1% potassium hydroxide, and trace of silica.
B Has granule sizes of 4–8 mesh.
C Loses about 30% of its weight when worn out.
D Produces heat of neutralization of up to 60°C.
E Should not be used with trichloroethylene.

TTFTT
B This size provides optimal balance between the surface area of the granules and the dead space between them.
C Soda lime gains about 30% of its weight (rather than lose) when worn out.
E Hot alkaline conditions may decompose trichlorethylene to toxic substances such as phosgene which may cause cranial nerve palsies.

4. Regarding Rotameter-type flowmeters:

A Density of the gas affects flow more at high flows.
B Viscosity of the gas affects flow more at low flows.
C The pressure difference across the bobbin is variable.
D Inaccuracies may be caused by a build up of static electricity.
E The flow meter reading is correct regardless of the type of gas flowing through it.

TTFTF

A,B At low flows, the gap between the bobbin and inner wall of the tube is narrow and long, therefore, the flow is more of a laminar type through a tube. At higher flows, with the bobbin at the top end of the Rotameter tube, the gap is wide and short, therefore, the flow is more of a turbulant type through an orifice.

C The pressure difference across the bobbin remains constant.

D,E There are a number of causes of inaccuracies including the build-up of static electricity, dirt on the bobbin, the flowmeter not being vertical and putting a different gas through the flow-meter to the one it was calibrated for.

5. The following statements are true:

A At constant temperature, the volume of gas varies inversely with its pressure.

B At constant pressure, the volume of gas varies directly with its temperature.

C At constant volume, the pressure of gas varies directly with its temperature.

D In a mixture of gases, the pressure exerted by each gas is the same as that which it would exert if it alone occupied the container.

E At same temperature and pressure, equal volume of gases contain equal number of molecules.

TTTTT

A This is Boyle's law.

B This is Charles' law.

C This is the third gas law.

D This is Dalton's law of partial pressures.

E This is Avogadro's hypothesis. Remember also Avogadro's number; at standard temperature and pressure, 1 g MW of any gas occupies a volume of 22.4 l.

6. One atmosphere pressure is approximately equivalent to:

A 100 kPa units.

B 1 kg per square centimeter (kg/cm^2).

C 15 lb per square inch (psi).

D 800 cm of water (cm H_2O).

E 1 bar.

TTTFT
A,B,C,D,E One atmosphere pressure is equivalent to: 1 bar, 100 kPa, 1 kg/cm^2, 15 psi, 100 kPa, 1000 cm H_2O, 760 mmHg or 760 torr.

7. The Manley ventilator:

A May be regarded as a constant flow generator.
B Changes in fresh gas flow cause changes in minute ventilation and ventilation rate.
C Rebreathing is determined by the amount of fresh gas flow.
D Is well suited for asthmatic patients.
E Is suitable for children of all ages.

FTFFF
The Manley ventilator is a time cycled minute volume divider. Preset fresh gas flow and volume determine minute ventilation and ventilation rate. The ventilator does not allow rebreathing and the only way to achieve that is by introducing dead space between the ventilator circuit and the patient. It is classified as a weak ventilator, unable to generate constant flow or high inflation pressure. It is not suitable for infants and small children.

8. Laminar flow of gas or liquid through a tube is directly proportional to:

A Its density.
B Its viscosity.
C The pressure difference across the tube.
D The fourth power of the radius of the tube.
E The length of the tube.

FFTTF
Laminar or parabolic flow is directly proportional to the pressure difference across the tube and the fourth power of the radius of the tube, and inversely proportional to the length of the tube and viscosity of gas or liquid. Turbulant or orifice flow is directly proportional to the second power of the radius and the square root of the pressure, and inversely proportional to square root of the density of gas or fluid.

9. Nitrous oxide:

A Has a high blood/gas solubility coefficient.
B Supports combustion.

C Is manufactured from ammonium nitrate.
D Impurities may be detected by moistened starch-iodine paper.
E Is stored in cylinders which when full have a pressure of 137 bar.

FTTTF
Nitrous oxide has a low blood/gas solubility coefficient, resulting in a rapid onset of action. Though non-flammable nitrous oxide will support combustion. Nitrous oxide is produced by heating ammonium nitrate and impurities, higher oxides of nitrogen may be detected using moistened starch-iodine paper. The nitrous oxide cylinder when full has a pressure of 54 bar.

10. Where kg = kilogram, N = Newton, m = metre, Pa = pascal, s = second and J = joule, the following are true:

A kg is a basic SI unit of mass.
B N is a derived SI unit of force.
C N/m^2 is equivalent to Pa.
D m/s is a unit of acceleration.
E Watt = J/s.

TTTFT
D m/s is a unit of velocity. Acceleration, the rate of change of velocity, has a unit of m/s^2.

11. The following equations are true:

A Force = mass × acceleration.
B Weight = mass × gravity.
C Work = force × distance.
D Power = work/time.
E Pressure = force × area.

TTTTF
A Force (N) = mass (g) × acceleration (m/s^2).
   Remember $N = g.m/s^2$.
B Weight = mass × gravity.
C Work = force × distance.
D Power (Watt) = work per time (J/s).
E Pressure = force/area (N/m^2).

12. Critical temperature (CT):

A Is the temperature above which gas cannot be liquefied.

B Is the temperature at which a gas liquefies under critical pressure.
C Of oxygen is −118°C.
D Of Entonox is 4°C.
E Of water is 100°C.

TTTFF
A,B Generally speaking, the higher the temperature of a given gas, the higher the pressure required to liquify it. At the CT, a minimum pressure called 'critical pressure' is required to liquify it. Above the CT no pressure (however high) can liquify it.
D CT of Entonox is −7°C.
E CT of water is 400°C.

13. The following statements are true:

A Kelvin (K) is the SI unit of temperature.
B 273 K is approximately equivalent to 0°C.
C Specific heat capacity is the amount of heat required to increase the temperature of 1 kg of substance by 1°C.
D The heat capacity of a substance is its specific heat capacity multiplied by its mass.
E Specific heat capacity of gases is smaller than that of liquids.

TTTTT
A,B Kelvin (K) is the SI unit of temperature. The lowest possible temperature is 0 K, which is equivalent to −273°C. 273 K is equivalent to 0°C.

14. Regarding medical gases:

A Cylinder size B is larger than E.
B The weight of a size E cylinder when empty is nearer to 5 kg than 10 kg.
C Oxygen cylinders are coloured black with white shoulders.
D Nitrous oxide cylinders are coloured blue with white shoulders.
E In the UK, oxygen, nitrous oxide and air theatre terminal outlets (of pipelines) are coloured white, blue and white/black, respectively.

FTTFT
A Cylinders of medical gases are named alphabetically from small to large: B, C, D, E, F, AF, G, J. Note there is no A. The only cylinder made in size B is for cyclopropane (coloured

orange). Size E cylinder is the size commonly used on the anaesthetic machine.

B The weight of size E cylinder when empty is 5.4 kg.

C,D Oxygen cylinders are coloured black with white shoulders. Nitrous oxide cylinders are coloured blue with blue shoulders. Entonox cylinders are coloured blue with blue and white quartered shoulders. Air cylinders are coloured grey with white/black quartered shoulders.

15. The solubility of a gas in a liquid:

A Increases with increasing temperature.
B Is dependent on the partial pressure of the gas.
C Depends upon Henry's law.
D Depends on the type of liquid involved.
E Depends upon Charles' law.

FTTTF

A The solubility of a gas in a liquid decreases with increasing temperature.

B,C It also depends upon the partial pressure of the gas according to Henry's law.

D The type of liquid involved influences the solubility.

E Charles law states that 'at constant pressure, the volume of gas varies directly with its temperature'.

Clinical anaesthesia (10)

1. Concerning artificial ventilation:

A IPPV reduces venous return.
B IPPV reduces central venous pressure (CVP).
C PEEP reduces alveolar dead space.
D PEEP reduces venous return.
E The use of NEEP (negative end expiratory pressure) is obsolete.

TFFTT

A,B IPPV increases intrathoracic pressure, reduces venous return and may falsely increase the CVP.

C,D PEEP increases intrathoracic pressure, reduces venous return, improves oxygenation by reducing the shunt, but does not reduce alveolar dead space.

E NEEP can cause closing of the alveoli, atelectasis and collapse.

2. Recognized complications of massive blood transfusion are:

A   Hypercalcaemia.
B   Hypomagnesaemia.
C   Hypokalaemia.
D   Fat embolism.
E   Hypothermia.

FFFFT

A   Citrate intoxication and hypocalcaemia rather than hyper-
    calcaemia.
C   Stored blood has high plasma K level due to low pH and hae-
    molysed RBCs. This may cause hyperkalaemia.
D   Air embolism not fat embolism.

3. Concerning tests of coagulopathy:

A   Prothrombin time (PT) or INR are appropriate for monitoring
    warfarin therapy.
B   Partial thromboplastin time (PTT) is appropriate for monitor-
    ing heparin therapy.
C   Activated clotting time (ACT) is an appropriate monitor for
    intraoperative heparin therapy.
D   ACT normal range is 200–400 s approximately.
E   Hiss test is used to detect capillary disease.

TTTFT

A   PT and its ratio INR are sensitive to factors of the extrinsic
    pathway (especially factor 7) which are vitamin K dependent
    factors and therefore affected by warfarin therapy.
B   PTT is sensitive to factors of the intrinsic pathway, hence its
    suitability for monitoring heparin therapy.
C,D ACT is an appropriate test of heparin therapy in the peri-
    operative period because it is simple, quick and reasonably
    accurate. Its normal range is 75–150 s. Prolongation of this
    time is proportional to the dose of heparin. ACT of more
    than 250 s has been shown to be adequate for cardiac surgery;
    however, ACT of 400 s or more is generally used for this
    purpose.
E   In capillary disease, petechiae may be demonstrated when a
    tourniquet is inflated around the upper limb.

4. During cardiopulmonary resuscitation:

A   Dilated pupils usually indicate neurological damage.

B Intravenous adrenaline acts mainly by direct cardiac stimulation.
C Administration of calcium is valuable in the treatment of asystolic arrest.
D 10 ml of 10% calcium gluconate is as effective as 10 ml of 10% calcium chloride.
E Calcium ions should not be given to an intravenously running $NaHCO_3$ infusion.

FFFFT
A Dilated pupils are common due to high adrenaline levels (produced endogenously or given exogenously to the patient during resuscitation).
B The main beneficial effect is now believed to be an increase in SVR, therefore more effective CPR.
C Adrenaline is a first choice drug in asystole. Calcium ions may have a place in EMD.
D The gluconate is one-third as effective as the chloride, and also slower acting.
E $CaCO_3$ will precipitate.

5. Concerning internal jugular vein cannulation:

A Air embolism is a recognized complication.
B Compared to the left side, the right vein is more in line with the superior vena cava.
C Compared to the left side, the dome of the pleura is lower on the right side (i.e. probably less likely to be injured).
D Puncture of the thoracic duct is more likely when cannulating the right side.
E Horner's syndrome is one of the common complications.

TTTFF
A This is due to the low or sometimes negative pressure in central veins. To minimize air embolism, the procedure is carried out in 10–15 degrees head down tilt position. Also, the cannula should not be left open to air at any time.
B,C,D Cannulation of the right internal jugular vein is preferred because the right vein is more in line with the superior vena cava, the dome of the pleura is lower on the right side, and the thoracic duct is absent on the right.
E This is one of the complications of trans or inter-scalenus brachial plexus block, when some of the local anaesthetic may escape to the stellate ganglia. This may happen here if local

anaesthetic was used and infiltrated deeply near the stellate ganglia!!

6. Incidence of difficult intubation is increased in:

A Pierre Robin and Treacher Collins syndromes.
B Rheumatoid arthritis.
C Late pregnancy.
D Edentulous patients.
E Children aged 5–10 years.

TTTFF

A These two syndromes are associated with micrognathia, retro-gnathia and macroglossia with difficulty in airway maintenance and intubation.
C Factors contributing to difficult intubation are facial/oro-pharyngeal oedema, possibly macroglossia, large breasts, full dentition, and the conditions of rapid sequence induction with cricoid pressure due to the risk of aspiration.
D This may make laryngoscopy and intubation easier.
E Intubation is not difficult in children of this age; however, neo-nates and small infants require special skill and experience.

7. Difficult intubation is associated with:

A Small mandible.
B Receding jaw.
C Long thyromental distance.
D Temperomandibular joint syndrome.
E Large breasts.

TTFTT

C Difficult intubation is associated with short (rather than long) thyromental distance. Also associated with short sternomental distance.
E This makes difficult the introduction of the laryngoscope. Polio-blade laryngoscope may be useful in this situation. Also, short handle or variable angle laryngoscopes may be used.

8. In malignant hyperpyrexia susceptible (MHS) patients and when anaesthesia is necessary, the following anaesthetic agents must not be used:

A Thiopentone.
B Suxamethonium.

C Isoflurane.
D Atracurium.
E Bupivacaine.

FTTFF
In MH the following drugs must be avoided; inhalational anaesthetics such as halothane, enflurane, isoflurane, cyclopropane and ether (N_2O is probably low risk), depolarizing muscle relaxants such as suxamethonium, and phenothiazines in general. If anaesthesia is necessary then a choice may be made from the following list of low risk drugs; benzodiazepines such as diazepam, opiates, e.g. fentanyl, thiopentone or propofol, non-depolarizing muscle relaxants such as atracurium and vecuronium, bupivacaine of the local anaesthetics, and of course 100% oxygen.

9. Concerning a 12-lead ECG:

A Inverted P and QRS waves in lead 1 do not occur unless the leads are connected wrongly.
B A right bundle branch block (BBB) is more serious than a left BBB.
C PR and QRS intervals do not normally exceed 0.21 and 0.11 s, respectively.
D QT interval is inversely related to heart rate.
E Q waves in leads I, II, aVL or aVF of greater than 3 mm in depth or greater than one-quarter of the height of ensuing R wave are abnormal.

FFTTT
A This may occur in dextrocardia.
B Left BBB is commonly associated with significant cardiac disease, whilst right BBB may not be of clinical significance.
C PR of longer than 0.21 indicates first degree heart block, and QRS of longer than 0.11 s indicates interventricular conduction block, e.g. bundle branch block or abnormal conduction pathway, e.g. ventricular rhythm or ectopics.
D QT interval shortens with increases in heart rate and vice versa.
E These are the criteria for abnormal Q waves.

10. Concerning complications of brachial plexus block:

A Pneumothorax is more likely to occur with the supraclavicular approach than the interscalenus approach.

B Horner's syndrome is more likely to occur with the supraclavicular approach than the interscalenus approach.
C Phrenic nerve palsy is more likely to occur with the supraclavicular approach than the interscalenus approach.
D Intravascular injection is less likely to occur with the axillary approach than the supracalvicular or interscalenus approach.
E The use of bilateral supraclavicular or interscalenus brachial plexus block is safe provided that the maximum recommended dose of the local anaesthetic is not exceeded.

TFFFF
D Intravascular injection is a recognized complication of axillary approach. The injection is made perivascular and into the axillary sheath. Aspiration of blood should be checked at intervals during the injection or every time the needle is moved.
E Not only the maximum dose of local anaesthetic matters here, but also the risk of pneumothorax/phrenic nerve palsy bilaterally.

Statistics (5)

1. The following are non-parametric statistical tests:

A Chi-square test.
B Student's *t*-test.
C Willcoxon Rank tests.
D Analysis of variance.
E Mann–Whitney *U*-test.

TFTFT
A,C,E Examples of non-parametric tests are; Chi-square test, the sign test, Willcoxon signed rank test, Wilcoxon rank sum test, and Mann–Whitney *U*-test.
B,D Student's *t*-test and analysis of variance are parametric tests. Note that 'Kruskall–Wallis' may be regarded by some as a non-parametric version of analysis of variance.

2. Concerning probability:

A *P* value of less than 0.05 is usually regarded as significant.
B *P* value of less than 0.01 is usually regarded as highly significant.
C The choice of a *P* value for significance will affect the number of false positive and false negative errors.

D *P* value of 0.1 means a 1 in 10 chance that the result could have happened by chance.

E *P* value is suitable for parametric tests and not suitable for non-parametric tests.

TTTTF

C Choosing high or low *P* values result in an increase in false positive or false negative errors, respectively.

E It is suitable for both parametric and non-parametric tests.

3. In a normal (Gaussian) distribution:

A The median is the numerical value that is exactly in the middle.

B The mode is the most common numerical value.

C The mean and the median are identical.

D 95% of the population fall within one standard deviation on either side of the mean.

E Student's *t*-test is a suitable instrument for statistical analysis.

TTTFT

D Two standard deviations on either side of the mean will include 95% of the population.

E Parametric tests (such as Student's *t*-test) are suitable for analysing data with symmetrical distribution.

4. Where SD = standard deviation and SE = standard error, the following statements are true:

A The mean is the sum of observations divided by their number.

B The variance is the average of squared deviations from the mean.

C SD is a measure of dispersion of data around the mean.

D SD is the square root of the variance.

E SE (or SD of the mean) is the SD divided by the number of observations in the sample.

TTTTF

E This is the SD divided by the square root of the number of observations in the sample.

5. Parametric tests are used in the following cases:

A Data to be analysed have a normal distribution.

B Data are of nominal scale of measurement (e.g. blood groups).

C Data are of ordinal scale of measurement (e.g. Apgar score).

D   Data are of interval scale of measurement (e.g. temperature).
E   Data are of ratio scale of measurement (e.g. haemoglobin level).

TFFTT
A   Parametric statistics require the demonstration or assumption that data sets are normally distributed.
B   Nominal scale of data have no underlying continuum, therefore cannot be used in parametric tests.
C   The Apgar score is a rank order variable. Hence, a non-parametric test is most appropriate.
D,E Yes, if one can show or assume a normal distribution of data.

MCQs (30 pharmacology, 30 physiology and biochemistry, 15 physics and clinical measurement, 10 clinical anaesthesia and 5 statistics)

1. Renal blood flow:

A   Is independent of autoregulation.
B   Is 15% of the cardiac output.
C   Can be measured using para amino hippuric acid.
D   A greater proportion of flow goes to the medulla than the cortex.
E   Is decreased by frusemide.

FFTFF
Renal blood flow is regulated by a well developed autoregulatory system. It is normally 20–25% of the cardiac output. Renal blood flow can be measured using para amino hippuric acid, which is effectively removed from the circulation on one passage through the kidneys. The cortex receives 92% of the total renal blood flow. Frusemide increases renal blood flow.

2. Cinchocaine:

A   Is a local anaesthetic.
B   Is a quinolone derivative.
C   Is used to detect atypical forms of pseudocholinesterase.
D   Is metabolized in the liver.
E   Is a constituent of EMLA cream.

TTTTF

The local anaesthetic cinchocaine is a quinolone derivative. In a 10^{-5} M solution it is used to detect atypical forms of pseudocholinesterase. In this context it is referred to by its American name, dibucaine. Cinchocaine is liver metabolized. EMLA cream consists of 2.5% prilocaine and 2.5% lignocaine.

3. The Chi-squared test:

A Is suitable only for non-parametric data.
B Does not require a normal distribution.
C Requires a number of individuals to be greater than 30.
D Requires calculation of the expected frequency of observations.
E Is more powerful than a *t*-test.

FTTTF

The Chi-squared test can be used for data on any scale. It is not necessary to have a normal distribution for this test. The total number of individuals should be greater than 30. The test involves calculation of an expected frequency of an observation. Power of a statistical test in medicine depends upon the measured difference between a type of treatment and a placebo rather than the type of statistical test used.

4. Cerebral blood flow:

A May be measured by the Kety method.
B White matter receives a higher proportion of blood flow than grey matter.
C Cerebral blood flow is 54 ml/100 g per min.
D Is dependent on autoregulation.
E Decreases during convulsions.

TFTTF

Cerebral blood flow may be measured by inhalation of subanaesthetic concentrations of nitrous oxide – the Kety method. Total cerebral blood flow is 54 ml/100 g per min, grey matter receiving around twice the blood flow of white matter. Autoregulation is prominent in the cerebral circulation. Cerebral perfusion greatly increases during fitting.

5. Oxygen may be measured with:

A A Severinghaus electrode.
B Mass spectrometry.

C Paramagnetic analysis.
D Raman spectroscopy.
E The fenum detector.

FTTTF
The Severinghaus electrode measures carbon dioxide tension and the Fenum detector uses a chemical indicator to detect carbon dioxide gas. All the remainder can be used to measure oxygen.

6. The monoamine oxidase inhibitors:

A Include phenelzine.
B Metabolism shows genetic polymorphism.
C React with tyramine to produce hypertensive crisis.
D Pethidine can be safely administered concurrently.
E Can cause postural hypotension.

TTTFT
The monoamine oxidase inhibitors (MAOIs) include phenelzine and tranylcypromine. They are liver metabolized by acetylation, which shows genetic polymorphism. MAOIs interact with tyramine present in foodstuffs such as cheese producing hypertensive crisis. Pethidine interacts with MAOIs to produce a potentially fatal interaction of hypotension and respiratory depression. A recognized side effect is postural hypotension.

7. In the use of beta blocking drugs:

A Labetalol has both alpha and beta blocking properties, the beta blocking properties predominating.
B Practolol causes oculo–mucocutaneous syndrome.
C Metoprolol is a beta-1 selective agent.
D The symptoms of hypoglycaemia may be masked.
E Caution should be exercised in heart failure.

TTTTT
Labetalol has both alpha and beta blocking properties, beta blocking properties predominating in a ratio of 3:1. Practolol is no longer used as it causes oculo–mucocutaneous syndrome, consisting of skin rashes, corneal ulceration and peritoneal fibrosis. Metoprolol is a beta-1 selective agent. The normal sympathetic responses to hypoglycaemia are blocked by beta blockers. The negative ionotropic effects of beta blockers mean that they should be used with extreme caution in heart failure.

8. Transfer of a drug across the blood placenta barrier is known to be influenced by:

A Molecular weight of the drug.
B Lipid solubility of the drug.
C Plasma drug–protein binding.
D Placental blood flow.
E Maternal plasma concentration/time curve of the drug.

TTTTT
A Molecular weights usually determine the size of drug molecules.
B Remember biological membranes are mainly lipid. Drug ionization is also dependent on its lipid/water solubility.
C Normally only the free drug can cross biological membranes.
E This is especially important when drugs are administered during labour.

9. Capnography:

A Reliably confirms tracheal intubation.
B Relies on the fact that carbon dioxide is paramagnetic.
C Utilizes mass spectrometry.
D Works on the principle that carbon dioxide absorbs infrared light.
E Can detect increases in dead space.

TFFTT
Capnography reliably detects tracheal intubation as the lungs are the only organ that produces carbon dioxide gas. Capnography uses an infrared analyser, gases with two or more atoms such as carbon dioxide absorb infrared light to varying degrees. Large increases in dead space can be detected by the capnograph, as they produce a large decrease in the amount of carbon dioxide produced by the lung.

10. When measuring respiratory function with a vitalograph:

A Forced vital capacity is independent of height.
B An FEV_1:FVC ratio is normally 75%.
C Decreased FEV_1:FVC ratio can indicate restrictive lung disease.
D The asthmatic patient has a low FEV_1:FVC ratio.
E Patients with chronic obstructive airways disease tend to have a normal FEV_1:FVC ratio.

FTFTT

Forced vital capacity (FVC) and forced expiratory volume in 1 s (FEV$_1$) are related to height, age, sex and weight. The normal FEV$_1$:FVC ratio is around 0.75 in normal subjects. A decreased FEV$_1$:FVC ratio indicates airflow obstruction rather than restriction. The asthmatic patient has airflow obstruction and hence a decreased FEV$_1$:FVC ratio. With restrictive lung disease the FEV$_1$:FVC ratio is normal or increased.

11. Clinical trials:

A   Increasing the numbers in the sample decreases the probability of a type I error.
B   The likelihood of a type I error is reduced by accepting statistical significance at a lower probability.
C   Randomization increases bias.
D   A single blind trial occurs when both the doctor and patient are unaware whether the patient is receiving treatment or placebo.
E   A cross-over trial is inappropriate for a small number of patients.

TTFFF

A type I error occurs when a difference between two treatments is found to exist by a trial but in actual fact does not exist. Risk of a type I error is reduced by increasing the numbers in the sample and accepting statistical significance at a lower probability. Bias may be reduced by randomization and blindness. Single blind trials occur when the patient is unaware of treatment or placebo. Double blindness is when neither doctor nor patient is aware of treatment or placebo. A cross-over trial occurs when each patient acts as his own control, this is useful in a trial with a small number of patients.

12. Glucose handling by the kidney:

A   In normoglycaemia glucose is effectively completely reabsorbed.
B   Has a transport maxima of 11 mmol/l.
C   The bulk reabsorption occurs in the proximal part of the proximal tubule.
D   Is a passive process.
E   Is linked to sodium reabsorption.

TTTFT

In normoglycaemia practically all filtered glucose is reabsorbed. Once the transport maximum (11 mmol/l) of glucose is exceeded, glucose appears in the urine. Nearly all reabsorption takes place in the proximal part of the proximal tubule; it is an active process and glucose reabsorption is via a glucose sodium co-transporter.

13. Malignant hyperpyrexia:

A Is associated with the central core disease.
B Is associated with the King Denborough syndrome.
C Propofol may be safely used.
D Can be triggered by pancuronium.
E Sodium bicarbonate is used in cases of fulminating malignant hyperpyrexia.

TTTFT

Both central core disease and the King Denborough syndrome are associated with malignant hyperpyrexia. Both propofol and pancuronium are safely used in malignant hyperpyrexia. Fulminating cases are associated with a severe acidosis secondary to release of lactate from the muscle. This may be treated using sodium bicarbonate.

14. Following transurethral resection of the prostate the following would raise suspicion of the TURP syndrome:

A Hypertension.
B Hypotension.
C Nausea and vomiting.
D Convulsions.
E High serum sodium.

TTTTF

The TURP syndrome results from the absorption of large amounts of irrigation fluid from the prostatic bed. Due to acute hypervolaemia, hypertension and bradycardia occur initially. Decompensation can then occur, resulting in hypotension and pulmonary oedema. The CNS signs of the TURP syndrome include nausea and vomiting and as the serum sodium falls to levels of around 110 mmol/l, drowsiness, convulsions and coma can occur.

15. The Lambert–Eaton myaesthenic syndrome:

A Is always associated with bronchial carcinoma.
B Gives rise to distal limb weakness.
C Muscle power decreases with exercise.
D There is a decreased quantal release of acetylcholine at the motor end plate.
E Patients show an increased sensitivity to nondepolarizing neuromuscular blockers and a normal response to depolarizing neuromuscular blockers.

FFFTF

The Lambert–Eaton myaesthenic syndrome is associated with bronchial oat cell carcinoma and certain autoimmune diseases including scleroderma and thyroiditis. It gives rise to a proximal limb weakness which improves on exercise. Studies have shown that there is a decreased quantal release of acetylcholine from the motor end plate. Patients show increased sensitivity to both depolarizing and nondepolarizing neuromuscular blockers.

16. The colon:

A Reabsorbs 50% of the water load of the chyme presented to it.
B Actively secretes sodium into the lumen.
C Absorbs potassium from the luminal contents.
D Produces a stool containing 10% bacteria.
E Is essential for life.

FFFFF

The colon reabsorbs 90% of the water present in its contents. It also reabsorbs sodium while actively secreting potassium into the lumen. The stool produced contains 30–50% bacteria. The colon is not essential for life.

17. Local anaesthetic toxicity:

A The highest plasma concentrations of local anaesthetic occur with epidural block.
B Symptoms of cardiovascular toxicity occur before symptoms of central nervous system toxicity.
C Hypercarbia and hypoxia potentiate the toxicity of local anaesthetics.
D Central nervous system toxicity is usually manifested initially by coma.

E Lignocaine is the agent of choice for the treatment of bupivacaine-induced ventricular fibrillation.

FFTFF
The highest plasma concentrations of local anaesthetics occur in ascending order: subcutaneous infiltration, brachial plexus block, epidural, intercostal nerve block. The central nervous system is more sensitive to local anaesthetics than the cardiovascular system. Acidosis, hypoxia and hypercarbia all potentiate the toxicity of local anaesthetics. CNS toxicity is initially manifest by excitatory phenomena (visual disturbances, tinnitus, fitting) as the inhibitory neurones are more sensitive to local anaesthetics. As the concentration increases, excitatory neurones became blocked leading to generalized CNS depression and coma. Bretylium is the agent of choice for treating bupivacaine-induced ventricular fibrillation.

18. The sulphonylureas:

A Include metformin.
B Chlorpropramide has a half-life of 36 h.
C Decrease gut glucose uptake.
D Increase pancreatic insulin release.
E Cause lactic acidosis.

FTFTF
Metformin is a biguanide. Chlorpropramide has a half-life of 36 h. The sulphonylureas act by increasing pancreatic insulin release and do not affect gut glucose uptake. The biguanides, especially phenformin, are associated with lactic acidosis.

19. Drugs affecting blood coagulation:

A Heparin and warfarin are active both in vivo and in vitro.
B Heparin is an acidic glycosaminoglycan.
C Warfarin disrupts only the intrinsic part of the clotting cascade.
D Heparin is reversed by protamine.
E Warfarin has a short half-life.

FTFTF
Heparin is active in vivo and vitro; warfarin is active in vivo only. Heparin is an acidic glycosaminoglycan. Warfarin has a similar structure to vitamin K and disrupts modification of factors VII, IX, X and thrombin. Heparin forms a complex with antithrombin

III which inactivates thrombin and inhibits factors IXa, Xa, XIa, and XIIa. Warfarin disrupts the intrinsic, extrinsic and common clotting pathways. The action of heparin is reversed by protamine. Warfarin has a half-life of around 40 h.

20. Dantrolene:

A Is active orally.
B Can cause liver damage.
C When given intravenously is dissolved with mannitol and sodium hydroxide.
D Is a neuromuscular blocker.
E Increases the release of calcium from the sarcoplasmic reticulum.

TTTFF
Dantrolene is active both orally and intravenously. It is given orally to relieve muscle spasm in conditions such as multiple sclerosis. Prolonged administration has caused liver damage. Dantrolene for intravenous use is presented as 20 mg powder, 3 g mannitol and sodium hydroxide which should be dissolved in 60 ml water. Dantrolene is a muscle relaxant, acting by reducing the release of calcium from the sarcoplasmic reticulum; it does not interact with the neuromuscular junction.

21. The following drugs are enzyme inducers:

A Phenytoin.
B Rifampicin.
C Omeprazole.
D Sulphonylureas.
E Warfarin.

TTFTF
Both warfarin and omeprazole are enzyme inhibitors while the others are inducers.

22. The normal ECG:

A The P–R interval is from the end of the P wave to the beginning of the QRS complex.
B The P–R interval is normally not greater than three small squares.
C The QT interval remains constant with changes in heart rate.

D The U wave represents atrial repolarization.
E The T wave is negative in lead aVR.

FFFFT
On the normal ECG the P–R interval is measured from the start of the P wave to the start of the QRS complex. It is normally three to five small squares. The QT interval is taken from the start of the QRS complex to the end of the T wave. It is lengthened in bradycardias and shortened in tachycardias. Atrial repolarization is obscured by the QRS complex.

23. The Clark electrode:

A Produces a voltage so a battery is not required.
B Measures oxygen tension.
C Hydrogen ions are produced.
D Has a silver anode.
E The presence of halothane artificially raises oxygen tension.

FTFTT
The Clark electrode is used to measure oxygen tension, it requires a voltage (and hence a battery) for current to flow. Oxygen combines with water at a platinum cathode producing hydroxide ions. The anode is silver/silver chloride. The presence of halothane artificially raises the oxygen tension.

24. Diathermy:

A Produces a current of low frequency which reduces the risk of ventricular fibrillation.
B To prevent burning at the patient plate there is a low current density.
C Bipolar diathermy does not require a patient plate.
D The heating effects of diathermy are directly proportional to the current.
E Bipolar diathermy should be used in preference to unipolar diathermy in the presence of a pacemaker.

FTTFT
Diathermy produces a current of high frequency which minimizes the risk of ventricular fibrillation. The heating effect of diathermy is increased with increasing current density, at the patient plate the current density is low due to the large surface area so heating effects do not occur. With bipolar diathermy the circuit is

completed with the forceps, hence there is no requirement for a patient plate. The heat produced is proportional to current squared. If a diathermy is used in the presence of a pacemaker it should be of the bipolar type.

25. Cerebrospinal fluid:

A Is yellow in colour.
B Normally its volume is 150 ml.
C Has a lower osmolality than plasma.
D Is formed in the arachnoid villi.
E A lumbar CSF pressure of 100 mm CSF would be considered to be in the normal range.

FTFFT
Cerebrospinal fluid is normally colourless; its volume is around 150 ml, 75 ml surrounding the spinal cord and 75 ml surrounding the brain. It has an equal osmolality to plasma. CSF is formed in the choroid plexus and reabsorbed in the arachnoid villi. Lumbar CSF pressure varies between 60 and 150 mm CSF.

26. Halothane:

A Is a trigger of malignant hyperpyrexia.
B Produces trichloroacetic acid as a metabolite.
C Is stable in sunlight.
D Causes a reduction in mucociliary function.
E Halothane hepatitis has a similar incidence in adults and children.

TFFTF
All volatile anaesthetics have been implicated in the development of malignant hyperpyrexia. The metabolism of halothane produces a number of compounds including bromide, chloride, and trifluoroacetic acid. Halothane is presented in amber coloured bottles to prevent decomposition by light. Halothane causes a dose-dependent reduction in mucociliary function. The incidence of halothane hepatitis is much higher in adults than children.

27. MAC for a volatile agent:

A Is increased with increasing age.
B Is decreased by hypercarbia.
C Is decreased by the administration of sedatives.

D Should be measured after about 15 min of administration of the volatile agent in humans.

E Decreases if intubation is the noxious stimulus rather than skin incision.

FFTTF

MAC decreases with increasing age and the concurrent administration of sedatives. It is unaffected by $PaCO_2$. MAC should be measured when end tidal, alveolar, arterial and brain tensions are in equilibrium, usually around 15 min. MAC is increased by about a third when the noxious stimulus is intubation.

28. The knee jerk reflex:

A Is due to stretching of the patella tendon.

B Is due to stretching of the quadriceps muscle.

C A gamma fibres form the afferent limb.

D Involves L1–L2.

E The afferent limb enters the spinal cord via the ventral root.

FTFFF

Stretching of the muscle spindle in the quadriceps muscle leads to stimulation of the afferent limb of this reflex arc. A alpha fibres enter the spinal cord via the dorsal root at level L3–L4.

29. Gastrin:

A Is released by chief cells of the stomach.

B Is found within the CNS.

C Mediates gastric hydrochloric acid secretion by increasing intracellular cAMP levels.

D Secretion is increased by vagal efferent discharge.

E The kidney plays a role in its metabolism.

FTFTT

Gastrin is produced by G cells in the gastric antrum. Gastrin is present within the CNS in both the pituitary gland and the medulla; its function here is not known. Gastrin increases gastric acid secretion by increasing intracellular calcium ions. The secretion of gastrin is increased by vagal discharge. It is primarily metabolized by the small intestine and the kidney.

30. MAC of a volatile agent:

A Is a useful estimate of anaesthetic potency.

B Decreases with increasing body temperature.
C Increases with increasing atmospheric pressure.
D The MAC of halothane is lower than the MAC of methoxyflurane.
E Is related to the lipid solubility of the volatile anaesthetic.

TFTFT
MAC is a useful estimate of anaesthetic potency. It increases with increasing body temperature. The phenomenon of increasing atmospheric pressure increasing MAC is known as 'pressure reversal of anaesthesia'. Methoxyflurane has a MAC of 0.2%, while the MAC of halothane is 0.8%. The potency of a volatile agent and hence MAC is directly related to its solubility in lipid.

31. Suxamethonium:

A Its action at the neuromuscular junction is terminated by pseudocholinesterase.
B Consists of two linked acetylcholine molecules.
C Raises intragastric pressure.
D May be used safely within 6 months of a stroke.
E Bradycardia may accompany a second dose.

FTTFT
There is no pseudocholinesterase within the synaptic cleft; the activity of suxamethonium here is terminated by diffusion. Suxamethonium consists of two linked acetylcholine molecules. During the fasiculations associated with suxamethonium intragastric pressure rises. Suxamethonium is associated with an increase in plasma potassium of around 0.5 mmol/l; however, in certain conditions there is a very large rise in plasma potassium. For this reason suxamethonium should not be used within 6 months of a stroke. Sinus bradycardia (and even asystolic arrest) accompany a second dose of suxamethonium. Atropine should therefore be given before a second dose.

32. Soda lime:

A Contains mainly sodium carbonate when fresh.
B Reacts with carbon dioxide endothermically.
C The optimum size of the granules is 1.5–5 mm.
D The chemical indicator Clayton Yellow turns from deep pink to off-white when exhausted.
E May be safely used with trilene.

FFTTF

Soda lime consists mainly of calcium hydroxide when fresh. It reacts with carbon dioxide exothermically. The optimum size for the granules is 1.5–5 mm. Clayton Yellow is a chemical indicator in the soda lime which turns from deep pink to off-white when exhausted. Trilene decomposes in hot soda lime to form dichloro-acetylene and phosgene which are neurotoxic.

33. The rate at which the alveolar fraction of volatile anaesthetic increases to its inspired fraction:

A Is increased by increasing ventilatory rate.
B Is increased by increasing cardiac output.
C Is increased by using a volatile anaesthetic with a high blood/gas solubility coefficient.
D Is faster with desflurane than halothane.
E Is decreased when nitrous oxide is administered concomitantly.

TFFTF

Increasing ventilatory rate increases delivery of anaesthetic agent to the alveolus. Increasing cardiac output increases the removal of anaesthetic from the alveolus opposing the rise in alveolar tension of the anaesthetic. Anaesthetic agents with a high blood/gas solubility coefficient have a high rate of removal into the blood, thus opposing the increase in alveolar fraction of the anaesthetic. Desflurane has a blood/gas solubility coefficient of 0.4, halothane 2.3. Concomitant administration of nitrous oxide ensures an increase in the alveolar fraction of anaesthetic agent. This is because removal of a large volume of nitrous oxide into the blood draws in increasing amounts of volatile anaesthetic into the alveolus. This is the second gas effect.

34. Striated muscle:

A One sarcomere is the area between two adjacent Z lines.
B The H band consists of actin alone.
C In the resting muscle actin is tightly bound to troponin I.
D Calcium binds to troponin C.
E Blood flow to resting striated muscle is in the order of 10 ml/100 g per min.

TFTTF

In striated muscle one sarcomere is the distance between two adjacent Z lines. Each H band consists of myosin alone and decreases in size when the muscle contracts. Muscle contraction is brought about by increased intracellular calcium which binds to troponin C; this binding weakens the binding of actin to troponin I which is present in the resting state, allowing tropomyosin to move laterally exposing actin binding sites to myosin. Resting striated muscle blood flow is 2–4 ml/100 g per min.

35. Thyroid hormones:

A Are polypeptides.
B Exert their effect by binding to plasma membrane receptors.
C Release is stimulated by thyroid stimulating hormone, a glycoprotein.
D Increase the metabolic rate.
E T_4 has twice the potency of T_3.

FFTTF
Thyroid hormones are iodinated derivatives of tyrosine. They exert their effect by binding to nuclear receptors. TSH stimulates the release of thyroid hormone and is a glycoprotein. The thyroid hormones increase metabolic rate. T_3 has four times the potency of T_4.

36. The following changes occur with the maternal respiratory system in pregnancy:

A Minute volume increases.
B Vital capacity decreases.
C $PaCO_2$ increases.
D FRC decreases.
E Dead space increases.

TFFTF
Increasing the minute volume results in a reduced $PaCO_2$. FRC decreases during pregnancy, and in late pregnancy when supine closing capacity exceeds FRC. Dead space and vital capacity remain unchanged.

37. Ketamine:

A Exists as optical isomers.
B Is less lipid soluble than thiopentone.
C Has bronchodilator properties.
D Emergence phenomena are more common in children than adults.
E Has analgesic properties.

TFTFT
The phencyclidine derivative ketamine has a chiral centre and therefore exists as optical isomers. It is five to ten times more lipid soluble than thiopentone. Ketamine has bronchodilator properties. The emergence phenomena associated with ketamine are more common in adults than children (and the elderly). Ketamine produces profound analgesia at a dose of 0.5 mg/kg.

38. Ketamine:

A Raises both the blood pressure and the pulse rate.
B Is useful in psychotics.
C Metabolism produces active metabolites.
D May be given intramuscularly.
E Has a high incidence of allergic reactions.

TFTTF
Unlike the other induction agents ketamine increases the blood pressure and heart rate secondary to sympathetic stimulation. Because of emergence phenomena, ketamine is contraindicated in psychotics. A metabolite of ketamine is norketamine, which is active. Ketamine may be given intramuscularly to produce hypnosis at a dose of 10 mg/kg. Like etomidate, ketamine is associated with a very low incidence of allergic reactions.

39. The jugular venous pulse:

A Large 'a' waves are seen with junctional rhythms.
B The 'y' descent follows the 'c' wave.
C The 'y' descent is caused by opening of the tricuspid valves.
D The 'c' wave occurs during isovolumetric contraction of the ventricle.
E The 'v' wave is absent during atrial fibrillation.

TFTTF
The 'a' wave represents atrial systole, and is therefore absent during atrial fibrillation. Large 'a' waves are seen when the atria contract against a closed tricuspid valve which can occur during junctional rhythms. The 'c' wave represents bulging of the tricuspid valve into the atrium during isovolumetric contraction of the ventricle. It is followed by a sharp 'x' descent, which is due to downward displacement of the tricuspid valve during ventricular systole. The 'v' wave is due to a build-up of blood in the right atrium when the tricuspid valve is closed. Finally, the 'y' descent

occurs when the tricuspid valve opens and blood flows rapidly into
the ventricle.

40. Droperidol:

A May cause hyperpyrexia.
B Is a phenothiazine.
C Lowers blood pressure by alpha antagonism.
D Speeds gastric emptying.
E May produce extrapyramidal symptoms.

TFTFT
Droperidol, a butyrophenone has been implicated in the malignant
neuroleptic syndrome (a syndrome involving hyperpyrexia). It is
an alpha blocker and therefore lowers blood pressure. Droperidol
does not affect gastric emptying, it is an antiemetic by virtue of
its antidopaminergic action on the central chemoreceptor trigger
zone. Butyrophenones can cause extrapyramidal symptoms.

41. Clonidine:

A Is an alpha-2 adrenergic antagonist.
B Decreases the requirement for neuromuscular blockers.
C Has been used historically as an antihypertensive.
D Reduces the pressor response to intubation.
E Reduces MAC of the volatile anaesthetic agents.

FFTTT
Clonidine is an alpha-2 adrenergic agonist. It will produce analgesia, sedation and hypnosis. Clonidine does not affect neuromuscular blockade. Clonidine has been used historically as an
antihypertensive agent. Administration of clonidine will reduce
both the pressor response and the MAC of volatile anaesthetic
agents.

42. Etomidate:

A Inhibits 11-beta-hydroxylase.
B Is useful for long term sedation in intensive care units.
C Is associated with a low incidence of nausea and vomiting.
D Is commonly associated with venous thrombosis.
E Is used at doses of 1–3 mg/kg for induction.

TFFTF

Etomidate produces dose dependent adrenocortical suppression by inhibition of 11-beta-hydroxylase and to a lesser extent 17-alpha-hydroxylase. It is contraindicated for long term sedation on intensive care units, as the adrenocortical suppression leads to death. Etomidate is associated with a high incidence of nausea and vomiting. It is used for induction at a dose of 0.2–0.3 mg/kg.

43. Methaemoglobinemia is reversed by:

A Glutathione
B Acetalinide.
C The enzyme NADH methaemoglobin reductase.
D Phenacetin.
E Methylene blue.

TFTFT

Methaemoglobinaemia is induced by: prilocaine, nitrites, sulphonamides, methylene blue, phenacetin and acetalinide. It is reversed by: the enzyme NADH methaemoglobin reductase (endogenous), methylene blue, ascorbic acid and glutathione. Note that methylene blue can work both ways, i.e. induce and reverse methaemoglobinaemia.

44. Concerning the benzodiazepines:

A They have muscle relaxant properties.
B Midazolam cannot be used as a sole induction agent.
C Site of action is the GABA receptor.
D Midazolam is water soluble at physiological pH.
E Both midazolam and diazepam are protein bound to a limited extent.

TFTFF

Benzodiazepines posess the following properties: anticonvulsant, hypnotic, sedative, amnesic, centrally acting muscle relaxants. For induction of anaesthesia midazolam alone may be used at a dose of 0.3 mg/kg. The site of action is the GABA receptor, increasing chloride influx into the neurones. Midazolam is lipid soluble at physiological pH, having a ring structure which opens at a pH below 4, making it water soluble in an acid medium. Both midazolam and diazepam are 95–99% protein bound.

45. Regarding pharmacokinetics:

A The units of clearance are mg/min.
B Alcohol obeys zero order kinetics.
C As the volume of distribution increases, the fraction of drug eliminated in unit time decreases.
D Salicylates may obey both zero and first order elimination kinetics.
E The fraction of drug eliminated in unit time (K_{el}) is directly related to its half-life.

FTTTF
A drug is usually eliminated by first order elimination kinetics, i.e. its rate of elimination is related to the fraction of drug present in the body, an exponential process. In zero order kinetics the enzyme systems are saturated so that drugs are eliminated at a constant rate, for instance alcohol and high dose salicylates. Low dose salicylates are eliminated by a first order process. Clearance of a drug is the volume of plasma completely cleared of drug in unit time, the units are l/min. The fraction of drug eliminated in unit time, $K_{el} = 0.693 \div t_{1/2}$.

46. Protein binding of drugs:

A Is always to albumin.
B It is only the unbound fraction that is liver metabolized.
C It is only the unbound fraction which can cross membranes to exert a pharmacological effect.
D Concomitant administration of warfarin and salicylates may potentiate the effects of warfarin.
E Thiopentone is over 90% protein bound.

FFTTF
Protein binding of drugs occurs predominantly to albumin. Certain drugs, however, are extensively bound to alpha-1 acid glycoprotein, such as bupivacaine and lignocaine. Propranolol has an extraction ratio of 78%. It is between 90 and 95% protein bound. The liver must therefore be actively removing it from its plasma protein binding sites. It is the unbound fraction of drug that is able to cross membranes and exert a pharmacological effect. Drugs that are extensively protein bound (warfarin, phenytoin, tolbutamide) may be displaced from their binding sites by other drugs that are extensively protein bound, e.g. salicylates. Thiopentone is 85% protein bound.

47. Diuretics:

A   Mannitol is actively secreted into the proximal tubule.
B   Mannitol is useful in the treatment of raised intracranial pressure.
C   Acetazolamide produces a metabolic acidosis.
D   Amiloride is an antagonist of spironolactone.
E   High doses of bendrofluazide produce a marked diuresis.

FTTFF
Mannitol is filtered by the glomerulus and is not secreted or reabsorbed in the tubules. It is useful in the treatment of raised intracranial pressure. Acetazolamide is a carbonic anhydrase inhibitor, preventing sodium and bicarbonate reabsorption from the proximal tubule, this results in a modest diuresis. Loss of bicarbonate leads to a metabolic acidosis. Amiloride is a potassium sparing diuretic but it does not act specifically at the aldosterone receptor. Spironolactone, however, is a specific antagonist at the aldosterone receptor. Bendrofluazide, a thiazide diuretic, acts upon the distal tubule which accounts for 5% of the total sodium reabsorbed, so it is unable to produce a large diuresis regardless of any increase in dose.

48. In the distribution of data:

A   In a positively skewed distribution the mean is higher than the mode.
B   The mean and mode are measures of scatter.
C   The mode is the 50th percentile.
D   In a normal distribution the mode, median, and mean all have the same value.
E   In a normal distribution 68.3% of the variables lie within 1 standard deviation of the mean.

TFFTT
In a positively skewed distribution (i.e. a long tail towards the positive values), the mean has a higher value than the median which has a higher value than the mode. The mode is the variable with the highest frequency and the median is the 50th percentile. Both are measures of central tendency. In a normal distribution 68.3% of the sample is between +1 and −1 standard deviation from the mean. 94.45% of the sample is between +2 and −2 standard deviations of the mean. 99.73% of the sample is between +3 and −3 standard deviations from the mean.

49. Corticosteroids:

A   Bind to cytosolic receptors.
B   Mineralocorticoids cause hypokalaemia.
C   Glucocorticoids inhibit both B and T lymphocyte function.
D   Dexamethasone has predominantly mineralocorticoid effects with minimal glucocorticoid effects.
E   Beclomethasone is well absorbed across mucus membranes.

TTTFF
The corticosteroids exert their effects by entering cells and binding to cytosolic receptors, stimulating the synthesis of protein. Mineralocorticoids cause sodium retention, with increased loss of potassium resulting in hypokalaemia. Glucocorticoids inhibit both B and T lymphocyte function. Dexamethasone is a potent glucocorticoid with minimal mineralocorticoid effects. Beclomethasone is used topically as it penetrates mucus membranes poorly.

50. Morphine:

A   Is greater than 50% protein bound.
B   Can cause bradycardia.
C   Is commercially produced from papaver somniferum.
D   Has active metabolites.
E   Is a useful analgesic in biliary colic.

FTTTF
Morphine is 35% protein bound. It can produce a bradycardia by a direct stimulatory effect on the vagus nerve. Although morphine can be synthesized, it is commercially produced from papaver somniferum (the opium poppy). Morphine undergoes extensive liver metabolism, the major metabolite being morphine 6 glucuronide which is a potent 'mu' receptor agonist. Morphine causes sphincter of Oddi spasm and should be avoided in biliary colic.

51. Regarding statistical tests:

A   Statistical significance is taken as $P > 0.05$.
B   A statistically significant result indicates clinical significance.
C t-Tests are useful for parametric data.
D   The Mann–Whitney U-test is used for a non-Gaussian distribution.
E   Type II errors only occur when the null hypothesis is rejected.

FFTTF

Statistical significance is taken as $P < 0.05$; however statistical significance does not necessarily mean clinical significance. t-Tests are used with parametric data. The Mann–Whitney U-test is used with a non-Gaussian distribution. Type II errors occur when the null hypothesis is accepted.

52. The following are recognized changes in pregnancy:

A   Decreased lower oesophageal sphincter tone.
B   Increased MAC value for volatile anaesthetic agents.
C   Increased plasma levels of factors VII, VIII, and X.
D   Renal plasma flow rate remains unchanged.
E   Cardiac output increases solely by an increase in the stroke volume.

TFTFF

During pregnancy the gravid uterus shifts the position of the stomach, reducing the lower oesophageal sphincter tone which is often manifest as heartburn. During pregnancy the MAC of anaesthetic agents is lowered by 40%, the aetiology has not been definitively described. Pregnancy is a hypercoagulable state with increased plasma levels of factors VII, VIII, X and fibrinogen. Renal plasma flow rate increases rapidly during the first trimester, during the third trimester it returns to normal. Cardiac output increases due to an increase in both heart rate and stroke volume.

53. In the assessment of association between variables:

A   A scatter diagram is useful.
B   A positive correlation coefficient means that high values of one variable are associated with low values of the other variable.
C   A negative correlation coefficient means that high values of one variable are associated with low values of the other variable.
D   A correlation coefficient of ± 0.8 shows a strong correlation.
E   A correlation coefficient of ± 1.0 often occurs with biological variation.

TFTTF

A scatter diagram is useful in assessing the association between two variables. The association may be calculated as the correlation coefficient. Its value ranges from $+1.0$ to -1.0. With biological variation the extremes do not occur, a figure of ± 0.8 is considered to be a strong relationship. Positive correlation coefficients indicate that a high value for one variable is associated with a high value for the other variable. Negative correlation coefficients indicate that a high value of one variable is associated with a low value for the other variable.

54. Sickle cell anaemia:

A   Is due to an abnormality of the alpha chains of haemoglobin.
B   Is an autosomal recessive condition.
C   Sickledex testing distinguishes between heterozygous and homozygous forms.
D   The erythrocytes in patients with sickle cell trait cannot sickle.
E   Tourniquets are contraindicated.

FTFFT
The abnormality in sickle cell disease is replacement of valine by glutamic acid at position six of the beta globin chain. It is inherited as an autosomal recessive condition. The heterozygous and homozygous form are formally distinguished by electrophoresis of haemoglobin, and the sickledex test demonstrates sickling which can occur in both conditions. In sickle cell trait sickling can occur at oxygen tensions below 4 kPa. Tourniquets are contraindicated, as the resultant hypoxia and stasis will promote sickling.

55. The stomach:

A   Secretes bicarbonate.
B   Produces 2 litres of fluid in 24 h.
C   Hydrochloric acid is secreted from the cells that also secrete intrinsic factor.
D   Gastric emptying is increased by cholecystokinin.
E   After a total gastrectomy parenteral intrinsic factor is necessary.

TFTFF
The surface cells of the stomach produce bicarbonate. The total fluid output of the stomach in 24 h is 2.5 l. The gastric parietal cells secrete both intrinsic factor and hydrochloric acid. Cholecystokinin delays gastric emptying. After a total gastrectomy parenteral injections of vitamin B_{12} are required.

56. The muscle spindle:

A   Consists of both intra and extrafusal fibres.
B   The nuclear chain fibre is larger than the nuclear bag fibre.

C Muscle spindles are arranged in series with the surrounding muscle fibres.

D A gamma fibres are the efferent innervation to the muscle spindle.

E A delta fibres are the afferent innervation to the muscle spindle.

FFFTF
The muscle spindle consists of intrafusal fibres; extrafusal fibres are the contractile elements of the muscle unit. The nuclear bag fibre is larger than the nuclear chain fibre and these fibres are arranged in parallel with the surrounding extrafusal fibres. A gamma fibres provide the efferent innervation, while the afferent innervation is A alpha to both intrafusal fibres and A beta to the nuclear chain fibres.

57. Hemisection of the spinal cord at T10 leads to:

A A distal flaccid paralysis ipsilaterally.

B Contralateral impairment of temperature sensation.

C Contralateral impairment of proprioception.

D Ipsilateral impairment of two point discrimination.

E Bilateral impairment of pain sensation distally.

FTFTT
Hemisection of the spinal cord results in Brown–Sequard syndrome, which is characterized by an ipsilateral spastic paralysis due to sectioning of the corticospinal tract which decussates in the pyramids. Contralateral impairment distally of pain and temperature is due to sectioning of the anterolateral funiculus. Fibres entering this tract decussate at the spinal level of entry. Ipsilateral impairment of fine touch and proprioception occurs as fibres in the dorsal column decussate in the medulla.

58. Basal metabolic rate:

A May be measured using spirometry.

B Is higher in children than in adults.

C Is subject to diurnal variation.

D Is related to body surface area.

E Men and women have equal basal metabolic rates.

TTTTF
Basal metabolic rate can be calculated from the oxygen consumption which may be determined using an oxygen filled spirometer

and a carbon dioxide absorber. Children have a higher metabolic rate than adults. The basal metabolic rate is highest in the morning and declines at night. In humans there is a strong correlation between basal metabolic rate and body surface area. Men have a higher metabolic rate than women.

59. Concerning the ABO blood groups:

A   This is a reference to the antigenic properties of the erythrocyte plasma membrane surface proteins.
B   Group A has the highest frequency in the UK.
C   Antibodies to A and B antigens are predominantly of the IgM type.
D   A patient with the AB blood group may be safely given blood of group B.
E   The ABO antigens are located only on the surface of erythrocyte plasma membranes.

FFTTF
The ABO blood group refers to the antigenic properties of erythrocyte plasma membrane glycolipids. The frequencies of the ABO blood groups in the UK are O: 47%, A: 42%, B: 8%, AB: 3%. Naturally occurring antibodies to A and B blood groups are predominantly of the IgM type. Patients with the AB blood group may be given blood of A, B or AB type as they have no anti-A or anti-B antibodies. The ABO antigens are not confined to erythrocyte plasma membranes and are found in a number of body fluids and organs.

60. The anterior lobe of the pituitary gland:

A   Is derived from Rathke's pouch.
B   Produces ADH.
C   Produces FSH.
D   Has a portal blood system linking it with the hypothalamus.
E   Produces prolactin when stimulated by dopamine.

TFTTF
The anterior lobe of the pituitary gland is derived from an evagination of the roof of the mouth called Rathke's pouch. It produces the following hormones: thyroid stimulation hormone, adrenocorticotropic hormone, luteinizing hormone, prolactin and growth hormone. Pituitary release of prolactin is inhibited by hypothalamic release of dopamine into the portal blood system, linking it with the anterior lobe of the pituitary gland.

61. Regarding calcium homeostasis:

A Intracellular calcium is at a higher concentration than extra-cellular calcium.

B Plasma calcium is lowered by parathyroid hormone.

C Uptake of calcium from the gut is decreased by 1,25-dihydroxycholecalciferol.

D Plasma calcium is raised by calcitonin.

E Hypercalcaemia may present as abdominal pain.

FFFFT

The extracellular calcium concentration is in the order of 2 mmol/l and intracellular calcium is in the order of 10^{-4} mmol/l. Parathyroid hormone is released in response to a low plasma calcium. It raises plasma calcium by activating osteoclasts to release calcium and phosphate into the blood. 1,25-Dihydroxycholecalciferol is produced by successive hydroxylations of vitamin D. It increases the absorption of calcium from the gut. Calcitonin lowers plasma calcium by increasing calcium absorption into bones. Hypercalcaemia may present as abdominal pain.

62. The sodium–potassium pump:

A Moves two sodium ions out of the cell in exchange for three potassium ions into the cell.

B Is electrogenic.

C Is involved in maintaining the resting membrane potential.

D Does not affect cell volume.

E Is inhibited by cardiac glycosides.

FTTFT

The sodium–potassium pump moves three sodium ions out of the cell for two potassium ions into the cell. This leads to a net intracellular negative charge, and the pump is therefore electrogenic. The sodium–potassium pump is involved in maintaining the negative resting membrane potential, making it 10 mV more negative than it would be due to passive ion currents alone. The sodium–potassium pump also prevents cellular swelling. Inhibition of the pump increases the membrane potential in the direction of the chloride equilibrium potential, increasing intracellular chloride; to maintain electrical neutrality cations would have to enter the cell (mainly potassium), and this would increase the intracellular osmotic pressure leading to water entry and swelling. The sodium–potassium pump is inhibited by cardiac glycosides.

63. Cardiac innervation:

A   Parasympathetic fibres are uniformly distributed throughout the heart.
B   In the normal heart parasympathetic tone predominates.
C   Parasympathetic stimulation increases the membrane permeability to potassium.
D   A-V nodal conduction remains at a constant rate with increasing parasympathetic stimulation.
E   Very rapid stimulation will tetanize cardiac muscle.

FTTFF
Cardiac innervation is via the sympathetic and parasympathetic nervous system. Whereas the sympathetic innervation is uniformly distributed throughout the heart, the vagal nerves supply the right atrium, the sinoatrial node, and atrioventricular node, innervation of the ventricles is sparse. The totally denervated heart beats at a rate of 110 beats/min, while the normal adult heart beats at a rate of 60–80 beats/min, implying vagal tone predominates. Parasympathetic stimulation increases membrane conductance to potassium, thus slowing the rate of nodal conduction. Cardiac muscle cannot be tetanized.

64. The following have vasoconstrictor properties:

A   Thromboxane.
B   Angiotensin II.
C   Histamine.
D   Bradykinin.
E   Serotonin.

TTFFT
Thromboxane is released from platelets and has vasoconstrictor properties, it also increases platelet aggregation. Angiotensin II is one of the most potent vasoconstrictors known. Both histamine and bradykinin have vasodilator properties as well as increasing vascular permeability. Serotonin is found in high concentrations in viscera and platelets. It has vasoconstrictor properties as well as increasing platelet aggregation.

65. Recognized effects of laparoscopic surgery include:

A   Decreased airway pressure.
B   Shoulder tip pain.
C   Regurgitation.

D Decreased cardiac output.
E Increased $PaCO_2$.

FTTTT
Splinting of the diaphragm decreases compliance leading to an increase in the airway pressure. Shoulder tip pain is common; this is referred pain from irritation of the diaphragm by carbon dioxide gas. Raised intra-abdominal pressure increases intragastric pressure, which can overcome the lower oesophageal sphincter pressure leading to regurgitation. Increased intra-abdominal pressure reduces venous return leading to a reduced cardiac output. The high solubility of carbon dioxide leads to an increased $PaCO_2$.

66. Aldosterone:

A Is synthesized in the zona glomerulosa of the adrenal cortex.
B Is a peptide hormone.
C Promotes sodium reabsorption in the proximal tubule.
D Increases the amount of potassium lost in the urine.
E Is released by antidiuretic hormone.

TFFTF
This steroid hormone is secreted by the zona glomerulosa of the adrenal cortex. Aldosterone promotes distal tubule reabsorption of sodium by increasing intracellular mRNA. As a consequence of increased sodium reabsorption, potassium and hydrogen ions are lost in the urine. Antidiuretic hormone does not release aldosterone.

67. On moving from the supine to the erect position:

A Total peripheral resistance increases.
B The carotid and aortic bodies fire at an increased rate.
C Cardiac output decreases.
D Heart rate decreases.
E Levels of circulating renin and aldosterone increase.

TFTFT
On moving from the supine to the erect position there is a transient pooling of around 500 ml of blood in the legs alone. This results in a decreased venous return and hence decreased stroke volume and decreased blood pressure. The resultant decrease in blood pressure causes a decreased firing rate of the carotid and aortic bodies. This results in an increase in total peripheral resistance due to arteriolar vasoconstriction and an increase in the

heart rate compensating for a drop in cardiac output. The decrease in renal blood flow results in activation of the renin–angiotensin system.

68. The Valsalva manoeuvre:

A Initially blood pressure drops.
B Release results in an initial rise in blood pressure.
C Release results in a tachycardia.
D Sustained Valsalva manoeuvre results in increased total peripheral resistance.
E Is a useful bedside test for autonomic neuropathy.

FTFTT
The Valsalva manoeuvre, forced expiration against a closed glottis, results in a rise in intrathoracic pressure. This leads to a rise in left ventricular stroke volume and an initial rise in blood pressure. This is followed by a reduction in the left ventricular stroke volume as the raised intrathoracic pressure retards venous return. The reduction in left ventricular stroke volume leads to a drop in blood pressure which is compensated for by a tachycardia and an increase in total peripheral resistance. Release of the Valsalva manoeuvre raises left ventricular stroke volume, raising the blood pressure and resulting in a reflex bradycardia. In the presence of autonomic neuropathy there is no bradycardia following release of a sustained Valsalva manoeuvre.

69. Lung surfactant:

A Is a steroid.
B Is secreted by type II alveolar cells.
C Molecules consist of both a hydrophilic and hydrophobic pole.
D Helps keep the lung dry.
E Absence results in stiff lungs, fluid filled alveoli and atelectasis.

FTTTT
The principle component of surfactant is phospholipid. Surfactant is secreted by type II alveolar cells. Having both a hydrophilic and hydrophobic pole to the molecule, surfactant opposes the normal intermolecular attractive forces, thus lowering the surface tension. Reduced surface tension also lowers forces that pull fluid out of the capillaries. Stiff lungs, fluid filled alveoli and areas of atelectasis are components of the infant respiratory distress syndrome which is caused by absent or reduced surfactant.

70. Concerning tests of lung function:

A Helium dilution and whole body plethysmography always give the same result when measuring total lung capacity.

B The anatomical dead space is measured using Fowler's method.

C The functional residual capacity can be measured directly using spirometry.

D Transfer factor test involves the inhalation of carbon monoxide.

E Closing volume may be measured using the inhalation of 100% oxygen.

FTFTT

Helium dilution measures only the volume of the airways that communicate with the atmosphere, whole body plethysmography measures the total volume of gas in the airways. In conditions where gas trapping occurs such as emphysematous bullae, helium dilution will give a lower value of total lung capacity. The anatomical dead space is measured using Fowler's method, plotting nitrogen concentration against expired volume after inhalation of 100% oxygen. Functional residual capacity cannot be directly measured using spirometry. The transfer factor test measures airway resistance by inhalation of carbon monoxide. The closing volume can be measured using the exhalation of nitrogen gas.

71. Airway resistance:

A May be measured using whole body plethysmography.

B Is independent of lung volume.

C Is decreased by ketamine.

D Is increased by isoflurane.

E The major site is the terminal bronchioles.

TFTFF

Airway resistance is measured using whole body plethysmography. As lung volume increases, the calibre of the conducting airways increases, lowering airway resistance. Airway resistance is lowered by both ketamine and isoflurane, which are bronchodilators. The major site of airway resistance is the medium sized bronchi, the terminal bronchioles contribute less to airway resistance because of their very large number.

72. The following increase with age in an adult:

A   Compliance.
B   Closing capacity.
C   Total lung capacity.
D   Vital capacity.
E   Residual volume.

TTFFT
Lung compliance increases with age, this is due to decreasing lung elasticity. Closing capacity increases with age. Total lung capacity remains unchanged. Vital capacity decreases with a consequent increase in residual volume.

73. From the base to the apex of the lung:

A   Ventilation increases at normal tidal volumes.
B   The V/Q ratio increases.
C   At residual volume ventilation increases.
D   In hypovolaemic states the apex of the lung may contribute to the alveolar dead space.
E   The decrease in blood flow from the base to the apex is primarily due to hypoxic pulmonary vasoconstriction.

FTTTF
During normal tidal ventilation both ventilation and perfusion decrease from the base to the apex. Perfusion decreases proportionally more than ventilation, resulting in an increasing V/Q ratio from the base to the apex. At residual volume however, the apex of the lung ventilates better than the base. In hypovolaemic states the capillary pressure in the apex can be exceeded by alveolar pressure, preventing blood flow (zone one), resulting in an increased alveolar deadspace. The decrease in blood flow from the base to the apex is primarily due to the effect of gravity on the low pressure, high capacitance pulmonary vasculature.

74. Carbon dioxide transport in the blood:

A   Carbon dioxide is less soluble in the blood than oxygen.
B   The majority of carbon dioxide is transported as bicarbonate.
C   As bicarbonate diffuses out of the erythrocytes electrical neutrality is maintained by extrusion of hydrogen ions.
D   Removal of bicarbonate from the tissues is increased in the presence of deoxygenated haemoglobin.
E   The carbon dioxide dissociation curve is sigmoid.

FTFTF

Carbon dioxide is 20 times more soluble than oxygen in blood. It is transported as bicarbonate, dissolved and in combination with proteins. The majority is transported as bicarbonate. As bicarbonate diffuses out of the erythrocyte, electrical neutrality is maintained by an influx of chloride ions. Deoxygenated haemoglobin is a more effective proton acceptor than oxyhaemoglobin, facilitating the formation of bicarbonate; this is the Haldane effect. The carbon dioxide dissociation curve is more linear than the oxygen dissociation curve and does not plateau out.

75. The P_{50}:

A   For normal haemoglobin is approximately 3.6 kPa.
B   Is a useful measurement for comparing different haemoglobins.
C   Is the oxygen tension when the haemoglobin is 50% saturated.
D   Is increased with carbon monoxide poisoning.
E   Is unaffected by temperature.

TTTFF

The P_{50} is the oxygen tension when the haemoglobin is 50% saturated, it has a normal value of approximately 3.6 kPa. Shifts in the oxygen dissociation curve are reflected by changes in the P_{50}, thus it is used to compare different haemoglobin dissociation curves. Carbon monoxide poisoning shifts the curve to the left, lowering P_{50}. P_{50} is increased with increasing temperature, hydrogen ion concentration and 2,3-DPG levels.

76. The carotid bodies:

A   Are innervated by the vagus nerve.
B   The firing response to increases in $PaCO_2$ is linear.
C   Respond to a decrease in arterial pH.
D   Are essential for life in humans.
E   Have a blood flow of 2000 ml/100 g per min.

FFTFT

The carotid bodies are situated at the bifurcation of the common carotid artery and are innervated by the glossopharyngeal nerve. They respond to decreases in PaO_2, pH and an increase in $PaCO_2$. The response to decreasing PaO_2 is very non-linear, firing rate plotted against PaO_2 produces a hyperbola. The carotid bodies are not essential for life.

77. Regarding ascent to high altitudes:

A The fraction of oxygen present in the atmosphere decreases.
B The partial pressure of oxygen in the alveolus decreases.
C Initially a respiratory alkalosis occurs.
D During acclimatization the buffering capacity of the blood increases.
E During acclimatization levels of 2,3-DPG increase.

FTTTT
The fraction of oxygen present in the atmosphere remains unchanged with increasing altitude, although its partial pressure decreases. The hypoxia that occurs with high altitude causes hyperventilation, leading to a respiratory alkalosis. Continued exposure to high altitudes produces a number of compensatory changes including increased erythrocyte production leading to increased buffering capacity of the blood. 2,3-DPG levels also increase, facilitating oxygen unloading in the tissues.

78. Hypothermia results in:

A Increased cardiac output.
B Impaired blood clotting.
C Loss of consciousness at 28°C.
D Increased myocardial irritability and ventricular fibrillation.
E J waves on the ECG.

FTTTT
Hypothermia results in a decreased cardiac output due to decreased contractility and rate. Hypothermia impairs blood clotting, this is due to a defect in platelet function. Loss of consciousness occurs around 28°C. As the temperature decreases the heart becomes more irritable, ventricular ectopics appear and ventricular fibrillation can occur. On the ECG J waves are present.

79. Heat disturbance under anaesthesia:

A Hyperthermia is more common than hypothermia.
B The majority of heat loss is by convection.
C May be reduced by the use of heat moisture exchangers.
D Volatile anaesthetics impair the vasoconstrictor response to decreasing temperature.
E To maintain normothermia the theatre temperature should be 20°C.

FFTTF

Hypothermia under anaesthesia is far more common than hyperthermia, the majority of heat loss being by radiation. Ten per cent of heat loss occurs in warming and humidifying dry inspired gases; this loss is reduced by using heat moisture exchangers. The volatile anaesthetics all reduce the vasoconstrictor response to decreased temperature increasing the tendency to heat loss. For normothermia the theatre temperature should be around 23°C.

80. Boyle's law:

A States that the volume of a fixed mass of gas at a constant temperature varies with the absolute pressure.
B States that at a constant pressure the volume of a mass of gas varies directly with the absolute temperature.
C States that a given mass of gas at a constant volume, the absolute pressure varies with temperature.
D Applies to ideal gases.
E Refers to a fixed volume of gas.

TFFTF

Boyle's law applies to ideal gases and states that for a fixed mass of gas at a constant temperature, its volume varies inversely with the absolute pressure. Charles' law states that at a constant pressure the volume of a mass of gas varies directly with the absolute temperature. The third gas law states that a given mass of gas at a constant volume, the absolute pressure varies with the temperature.

81. Concerning electrical safety:

A Class I equipment is earthed.
B Class III equipment has an external power supply.
C Microshock can occur at currents below the threshold of conscious perception.
D Class III equipment requires an earth.
E To increase patient safety in theatre, the patient should be earthed.

TFTFF

In class I equipment the casing is earthed. Class II equipment is not earthed, all accessible parts are doubly insulated. Class III equipment has an internal power supply. Microshock can occur at currents in the order of 100 microamps. The threshold for conscious perception of electricity is 1 milliamp. Earthing the patient increases the risk of electric shock.

82. Critical temperature:

A Of oxygen is −119.5°C.
B Of a gas is the temperature at which it cannot be liquefied regardless of any increase in pressure.
C Is a constant for all gases.
D At this temperature the vapour pressure of a gas is known as its critical pressure.
E The critical pressure of oxygen is 50.4 atmospheres.

TFFTT
The critical temperature of oxygen is −119.5°C. It is the temperature above which a gas cannot be liquefied regardless of any increase in pressure. The critical temperature varies with the gas concerned. The critical pressure is the vapour pressure of a gas at its critical temperature; for oxygen it is 50.4 atmospheres.

83. The fuel cell:

A Measures pH.
B Has a gold mesh cathode.
C Produces hydrogen ions at the cathode.
D Has a lead anode.
E As a battery is not required it has an indefinite life-span.

FTTTF
The fuel cell is used to measure oxygen tension. At the gold mesh cathode, oxygen reacts with electrons and water to form hydroxide ions. The fuel cell has a lead anode. It produces a voltage so a power supply is not required. However, like a battery it has a finite life-span.

84. The likelihood of turbulent flow increases when:

A Reynold's number is above 1000.
B Velocity is high.
C Density is high.
D Diameter of the tube is low.
E Viscosity is low.

FTTFT
The onset of turbulent flow is likely when Reynold's number exceeds 2000. Reynold's number = linear velocity × density× diameter ÷ viscosity.

85. During laminar flow:

A Flow is proportional to the radius squared.
B Flow is inversely proportional to the length of the tube.
C Flow is proportional to the viscosity of the liquid.
D Flow is directly proportional to the pressure change.
E Flow is inversely proportional to the density of the fluid.

FTFTF
Laminar flow is given by the Hagen–Poiseuille equation:

$$\text{Flow} = \pi \times \text{pressure gradient} \times \text{radius}^4 \div \text{viscosity} \times \text{length} \times 8.$$

86. Regarding potential fire hazards in theatre:

A Cyclopropane is flammable.
B The combustion of ether may be associated with 'cool flames'.
C Nitrous oxide is flammable.
D Cyclopropane can form explosive mixtures in air.
E Anaesthetic proof equipment is constructed to be used in areas where nitrous oxide or oxygen are the oxidizing agents.

TTFFF
Cyclopropane is flammable in air and can produce explosive mixtures in oxygen. This is also true of ether, cool flames are associated with the combustion of ether in air, these occur when the ether concentration is at the upper limit of flammability, cool flames are at a lower temperature than normal flames and ether is only partially oxidized. Nitrous oxide is not flammable. Anaesthetic proof equipment is constructed for use where air is the oxidizing agent.

87. The stages of anaesthesia as described by Guedel:

A Were described in unpremedicated patients inhaling ether and air.
B During stage II there is pupillary dilatation.
C The carinal reflex is depressed at stage III, plane II.
D Stage III is also known as surgical anaesthesia.
E Stage IV is regularly encountered in modern anaesthetic practice.

FTFTF

In 1937 Guedel published his description of the clinical signs of anaesthesia. Patients were premedicated with morphine and inhaled ether and air. Four stages were described.

Stage I (analgesia): amnesia, analgesia, regular ventilation.

Stage II (delirium): excitation, pupillary dilatation, irregular ventilation.

Stage III (surgical anaesthesia): this stage has four planes:

Plane I regular ventilation, pupillary constriction, pharyngeal and vomiting reflexes depressed.

Plane II eyes become immobile with depression of the corneal reflex.

Plane III ventilation becomes diaphragmatic, the eyelid and corneal reflexes are absent.

Plane IV ventilation is totally diaphragmatic, pupillary dilatation occurs, carinal reflex is absent.

Stage IV overdose with impending cardiorespiratory arrest.

88. Intraoperative gas embolus:

A   Is a recognized complication of laparoscopy.
B   The central venous pressure rises while the pulmonary artery pressure drops.
C   Is sensitively detected using Doppler ultrasound.
D   Gas bubbles may be aspirated using a central venous catheter.
E   Patients should be placed in a steep head down tilt and turned to the right lateral side.

TFTTF

Venous gas embolus is a recognized complication of laparoscopy. Both the central venous pressure and the pulmonary artery pressure rise. Doppler is a very sensitive method of detection. Treatment includes the administration of 100% oxygen, aspiration of gas bubbles using a central venous catheter and placing the patient in Durant's position, left lateral side with a steep head down tilt. This position displaces gas bubbles from the right ventricular outflow tract.

89. The following can be associated with a difficult intubation:

A   Down's syndrome.
B   Pierre Robin syndrome.
C   Scleroderma.
D   Von Recklinghausen's disease.
E   Obesity.

TTTTT
Down's syndrome with a large tongue and a small mouth can make intubation difficult. Pierre Robin syndrome with micrognathia, posterior displacement of the tongue and mandibular hypoplasia make intubation difficult. The tight skin in scleroderma can reduce mouth opening. Multiple fibromas of the larynx and pharynx can make intubation difficult with Von Reckinghausen's disease. Obesity is well recognized to be associated with difficult intubation.

90. When performing subarachnoid block the following factors are true:

A   A sensory block to T3 results in sympathetic denervation of the heart.
B   A Sprotte needle produces a lower incidence of headache than a Quincke needle of the same gauge.
C   The spinal cord in adults ends at the lower border of T12.
D   For a TURP the upper level of the block should be T12.
E   Raised intracranial pressure is a relative contraindication.

TTFFF
During subarachnoid block the sympathetic block is always two or more dermatomes higher than the sensory block. The Sprotte needle has a pencil point which parts the dural fibres rather than cutting them. The Quincke tip needle has a cutting tip and hence the incidence of post dural puncture headache is higher with a Quincke tip. In adults the spinal cord ends at the lower border of L1. For TURP the upper limit of the block must be T10. Raised intracranial pressure is an absolute contraindication to subarachnoid block.

4

The viva section

The vivas are primarily a test of your knowledge. They are also a test of your ability to present your knowledge in a logical and clear way. You can't make up for lack of knowledge by good presentation. You can, however, with bad technique, leave the examiner without a clear idea of how good you are. That would be a disaster!!!! The purpose of this section is to help you sell yourself to the examiner and present what you know in such a way as to maximize your knowledge.

Leading up to the vivas, you must get yourself in the right frame of mind. Ask yourself questions and either get someone else to listen to you, or look at yourself in the mirror while answering. In fact, whenever you have a spare few minutes, e.g. on the toilet or in the bath, practise answering viva questions. There's nothing like going through the side effects of suxamethonium to concentrate the mind. At work nag people to viva you. It doesn't just have to be consultants. It is as important to practice talking as it is to read books. You will have read the books anyway for the written part of the exam. Whatever happens, don't read the books the day before your viva. You have more chance of winning the lottery than being asked a question about something you have read at the last minute. The day before the viva should be spent using your credit card, relaxing and concentrating on speaking slowly and clearly.

On the day of the viva you must look the part. This is a professional exam. It has rules by which you must abide. That means that even if you feel anti-establishment, don't dress like it. White socks are right out!!!!! (There is one examiner who fails everybody in white socks and slip-on shoes and quite rightly). Comb your hair etc. Better still, ask your mother to get you dressed!!!

When you arrive at the exam hall, don't talk to anybody. They will only try to put you off. When its your turn for the viva the game begins. Dry your sweat drenched hands on your clothes, and the men should check their flies. When you walk into the hall, you have to show the examiner that you are in control without being cocky. Walk up to your table with your head held up and not like a lamb to the slaughter, and try not to trip over anything. Greet your examiners with a 'good morning/afternoon' (check the time before you go in), and sit down. To avoid nervous flapping of your hands throughout the viva sit on them, or put them on your knees. Just don't wave them about. Don't slouch. Sit up straight. You're not in the pub, yet!!!!!

Make a point of turning your chair to face the first examiner. When the second examiner starts, turn your chair to face him. The examiner not asking the questions usually marks your answers. It's very hard, but try not to take a peek at what he's writing. When you're answering, look the examiner who has asked you the question in the eye. If you look at the wall behind him or at your feet, or cross your arms, he'll know he's got you on the run. Even if you don't know the answer, look him in the eye and tell him you don't know. Don't, whatever you do, be arrogant, and never argue with the examiner. You can disagree with him but always be polite.

While the examiner is asking you a question, look interested and listen. If you don't listen to him, you may well answer what you think he's asking rather than what he is actually after. When he's finished his question take a few seconds to compose yourself. Pauses always appear longer than they actually are. The first thing you say sets the tone for the rest of your answer. Tell the examiner what you do every day at work. Don't make things up or lie. If they ask you to pick up a piece of equipment and talk about it, choose one that you've seen before. You may laugh, but one of the authors chose a Touhy needle from amongst hundreds of pieces of equipment, and when asked how many epidurals he had done had to say 'none sir!!'. He got another chance and chose an enflurane filling key instead.

Questions can be of various types. Practice before the viva will help you recognize them on the day. Specific questions such as 'What is pKa?' require specific answers. With an open-ended question such as 'How does a pulse oximeter work?', try to start your answer with a definition. In this example you could say 'a pulse oximeter is a piece of monitoring equipment commonly used in anaesthesia and intensive care which non-invasively measures arterial oxygen saturation'. This not only makes you start at the beginning, but also gives you time to clear your thoughts and decide what to say next.

If possible, try to categorize your answer. So if the question is 'What are the causes of a patient going blue during a laparotomy?', divide your answer up into respiratory causes and cardiac causes. You can further divide the respiratory causes up into problems with the patient and problems with the equipment. Categorizing your answers allows you to tell the examiner what you are going to talk about and focuses your mind on specific aspects of a topic rather than having lots of thoughts rushing around in your head making your answer sound muddled.

Always mention simple things first, leaving the complicated stuff until as late as possible. In other words TRY NOT TO DIG A HOLE FOR YOURSELF TOO EARLY!!!!!!! Having said that, don't make the examiner work too hard to get the facts from you, it will just annoy him. So if the examiner asks you about Entonox, don't start by telling him about what happens when the cylinder gets too cold. This will lead you into discussions about the Poynting effect, gases versus vapours etc. and you would have missed the opportunity to tell him what you know. That is that Entonox is a 50:50 mixture of nitrous oxide and oxygen which is stored in blue cylinders with blue and white quartered shoulders and is used for . . . etc.

When you think you have answered the question, stop talking and make the examiner ask you another. If he just sits there, ask him if he would like you to say anything else. Always try to stay in control. One of the most important things is not to get flustered if you get something wrong. If you realize you've said something wrong or that you have missed something out, ask the examiner if you can start your answer again. Remember, that even if you are the next Sir Ivan Magill, you will reach a point where you will answer a question incorrectly or simply not know the answer. People always remember the things they get wrong and not the questions they get right and we are notoriously bad at assessing ourselves. When you've finished a question, forget it and get on with the next one. You are probably doing better than you think.

There are certain questions which have bells attached to them and come with flashing lights. You usually get one of these per viva. They have to be recognized and answered correctly and confidently. Examples are the bleeding tonsil, anaphylaxis, failed intubation drill and anaesthesia in a patient with a full stomach. You must have clear answers to these questions before you go in to the viva room. The viva should not be the first time you've ever thought about how to check an anaesthetic machine or what you would do if you failed to intubate someone. So, these questions need to be practised over and over again beforehand. Remember, if you kill someone in a viva you will fail.

With all these points in mind we will set out some viva questions, answering some of them and giving hints in a few, but leaving you to answer the majority. Use this section to practise talking and to learn the rules of the game.

To recap, the format of the vivas is as follows:

Viva 1 – 30 min

15 min on pharmacology and statistics.
15 min on physiology and biochemistry.

Viva 2 – 30 min

15 min on physics, safety, clinical measurement.
15 min on clinical topics.

1. Pharmacology and statistics

(a) What are the side effects of suxamethonium?

Common things should be mentioned first (hopefully you will not need to discuss the rarer aspects in depth):

e.g. myalgia, bradycardia, raised intra-ocular and intracranial pressure, hyperkalaemia, allergy

THEN

pseudocholinesterase deficiency, MH, dual block

The examiner may ask about any of the things you mention. If he decides that he wants to ask about pseudocholinesterase deficiency, there is nothing you can do about it. However, at least you will have mentioned the common things and scored some marks first!!!!

(b) Tell me about drug X?

If they ask you a general question about a drug, they are NOT solely asking you about its pharmacology. There are other aspects of drugs to discuss and score marks on. A recommended way is to have a logical sequence in which to discuss the drug:

(i)   DEFINITION.
(ii)   STRUCTURE.
(iii)   MANUFACTURE: e.g. manufacture of nitrous oxide.
(iv)   PRESENTATION.
(v)   USES.
(vi)   ROUTE OF ADMINISTRATION.

(vii) PHARMACOLOGY: mode of action, dose, onset time, duration of action, volume of distribution, half-life.

(viii) METABOLISM AND EXCRETION.

(ix) CLINICAL EFFECTS: drugs act on all the systems of the body – from the top down these are – brain, eyes, lungs, (allergy in here), heart, bowels, liver, kidneys, placenta, muscle, neuromuscular junction, skin (everything gives you a rash!!!).

(x)   SIDE EFFECTS.

(xi) CONTRAINDICATIONS.

For example, the question may be 'Tell me about morphine'.

Wrong answer:

Morphine is an analgesic which acts on mu receptors which are found in the spinal cord and thalamus . . . . . . FACTUALLY THIS IS NOT WRONG, BUT YOU MAY BE DIGGING A BIG HOLE FOR YOURSELF. WORSE STILL, YOU WILL NOT HAVE MENTIONED OBVIOUS AND UNCONTRO-VERSIAL FACTS.

Better answer:

- Morphine is a naturally occurring opioid analgesic drug. Its structure is . . . . (if you know the structure, and for the commoner drugs you should, ask the examiner if you can draw it for him. This not only wastes time, but will get you major Brownie points!!!).
- It is presented in clear ampoules containing 10 mg/ml, 50 mg/ml etc., stored at room temperature in the CD cupboard.
- It is used as an analgesic in both the acute and chronic pain setting.
- It can be administered orally, intravenously, via PCA pumps, intramuscularly, subcutaneously . . . . , epidurally, spinally, intra-articularly.
- The dose depends on the route of administration and the intensity of pain.
- The effects of morphine are: analgesia, sedation (BRAIN), constriction of the pupil (EYE), respiratory depression (LUNGS), vasodilation and bradycardia (HEART), constipation, nausea and vomiting (BOWELS), spasm of the sphincter of Oddi (LIVER), crosses the placenta (PLACENTA) and flushing, itching and a rash (SKIN).
- Its side effects are . . . .

- Its absolute contraindications are known allergy.
- Its relative contraindications are sleep apnoea.

Having mentioned the obvious, and scored easy marks all the way, you can't avoid telling the examiner the nitty-gritty, i.e. the mode of action, half-life, volume of distribution, metabolism and excretion.

(c) What is MAC?

This illustrates that you have to know your definitions, including pKa (we were asked it), half-life, volume of distribution, agonist, antagonist, tolerance, pH, etc.

By the way, MAC is 'the minimum alveolar concentration of a volatile anaesthetic vapour, delivered in 100% oxygen, which prevents purposeful movement in 50% of young ASA I and II unpremedicated adult patients in response to a standard surgical stimulus (1 inch skin incision)'.

You need to know what it is altered by, e.g. age, premedication, nitrous oxide etc., and the MAC values of the five commonly used anaesthetic vapours.

pKa is 'the negative log of the dissociation constant'.

(d) What drug do you use for . . . ?

CHOOSE A DRUG WHICH YOU KNOW ABOUT, NOT NECESSARILY THE ONE YOU USE!!!

Analgesia	Say morphine
Maintenance	Say enflurane not sevoflurane, which you don't know enough about
Raising blood pressure	BEFORE MENTIONING A DRUG, DEFINE BP = CO × TPR AND THAT CO = SV × HR. Then, depending on the cause, choose the most commonly used drugs, e.g. inotropes, vasoconstrictors.

(e) What is desflurane?

What are its properties?
Can it be used for an inhalational induction?
What is its boiling point?
What sort of vaporizer is required for its administration?
Why is the vaporizer heated?
Which other volatile anaesthetic vapour requires a heated vaporizer?

(f) What effects do anaesthetic drugs have on the eye?

Don't panic. Think logically and you'll be surprised how many things you will come up with. To buy yourself time, define what you are going to talk about and categorize your answer. For example, you could start by saying that the eye can be divided into several structures which can be affected by anaesthetic drugs. Start at the front of the eye and work inwards and don't forget that we use a wide range of drugs in clinical anaesthetic practice, e.g. atropine, adrenaline.

Answering the question like this will avoid rushing straight into a discussion about suxamethonium and raised intra-ocular pressure and anaesthesia in a patient with a penetrating eye injury. Lead the examiner the way you want to go.

(g) What is half-life?

Give an example of a drug with a short half-life.
Give an example of a drug with a long half-life.
What is the half-life of propofol?
Why is propofol used for day case procedures?

(h) How can diuretics be classified?

This is fair game. They can ask you about any drug your patient may be on when you anaesthetize them or that you may use in ITU. You need to know the basics about these drugs.

(i) In what ways do drugs act in the body?

Classify.

(j) How are anaesthetic drugs metabolized/excreted?

(k) What do you understand about volume of distribution?

Give an example of a drug with a large volume of distribution.
Give an example of a drug with a small volume of distribution.
How is volume of distribution related to clearance of a drug?

(l) What do you understand by partition coefficients?

How does the blood/gas partition coefficient relate to speed of induction and recovery?
How does the oil/gas partition coefficient relate to MAC?

2. Physiology and biochemistry

(a) What is functional residual capacity (FRC)?

This is a good opportunity for you to draw a diagram of lung volumes. Remember to label all your diagrams. When you draw a graph, label the axis.

> What factors affect FRC?
> How is FRC measured?

(b) What is dead space?

> Define this. Remember there are two sorts of dead space, anatomical and physiological.
> Describe Fowler's method for measuring anatomical dead space.
> Describe the characteristics of the waveform.
> What is the final increase in measured nitrogen due to?
> Derive Bohr's equation describing physiological dead space.
> What is the normal value of VD/VT?
> What disease processes increase dead space?
> What will happen to expired CO_2 if dead space increases?

(c) What is the oxygen cascade?

> What is the effect of altitude on the oxygen cascade?

(d) Derive the alveolar gas equation.

A lot of people get asked this. It is fair game and gets you easy marks if you practise beforehand. You must also know what the implications of the equation are.

> What are the causes of hypoxia?
> What is shunt?
> Derive the shunt equation.
> What determines the partial pressure of alveolar carbon dioxide?
> What factors affect the respiratory quotient?

(e) What do you understand by ventilation perfusion mismatch in the lung?

> Why does it occur?
> Draw the graph relating alveolar pCO_2 to pO_2.
> What are the V/Q ratios at the apices and bases of the lung in an erect person?

(f) Plot the oxygen dissociation curve.

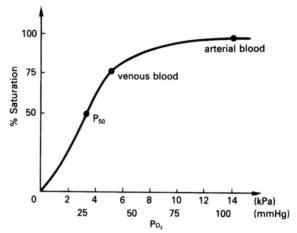

Figure 4.1 (Reproduced from Yentis, Hirsch and Smith (1995) *Anaesthesia A–Z* by permission)

Label the axis with units. Talk while you draw. Don't just draw an 'S' shaped curve. You have to indicate points through which the line goes. There are four of these (Figure 4.1).

What factors cause it to be shifted?
Why is this physiologically advantageous?

(g) What is lung compliance?

What is the compliance of the normal lung?
What physiological factors or disease states effect lung compliance?

(Don't forget to mention that in the clinical setting chest wall compliance may be abnormal although lung compliance may be normal.)

(h) Draw the action potential in the ulnar nerve.

The ulnar nerve is a mixed motor and sensory nerve. Don't simply draw the action potential in a single nerve fibre. Your drawing must take into account the various different fibres which make up a mixed motor/sensory nerve. Label the diagram.

(i) What factors contribute to intracranial pressure?

What are the causes of raised intracranial pressure?

How are pCO_2, pH, pO_2 and blood pressure related to intracranial pressure?
How can raised intracranial pressure be reduced?

(j) How do you smell?

One of the authors was asked this and was prepared for it as this question was asked a lot the year he took it. The examiners also asked about the other senses, i.e. taste, hearing, seeing. It's worth knowing about these in brief detail so as not to be phased if they ask you.

(k) Draw the action potential in cardiac muscle.

As you draw the different phases, describe the ionic shifts responsible for the potential changes you draw. It's always a good idea to talk as you draw. REMEMBER TO DRAW AND LABEL AXES.

How does the action potential in cardiac muscle differ from the action potential seen in a nerve?
How do positive and negative inotropes affect the cardiac muscle action potential?

(l) Draw the pressure waveform you would expect to see after inserting a central venous line into the right internal jugular vein.

Draw the a, v and c waves. Describe, as you draw, when in the cardiac cycle these waves occur.

What is the normal pressure in the right atrium?
What are the pressures in the other chambers of the heart and pulmonary and systemic vascular tree?

(m) Draw a capillary loop. What are the pressures exerted throughout this loop?

What is colloid oncotic pressure?
What is osmotic pressure?
What are the pressures in the lung capillary? What happens in the lung capillary loop in heart failure?
What are the pressures in a glomerular capillary?

(n) What is cardiac output?

This question can be a gift or a disaster. Define cardiac output (mentioning the units it is measured in) first. Then try to guide the examiner into something you know about like what factors affect cardiac output. Try to avoid going straight into a discussion about how you would measure it before mentioning the easier stuff.

How would you measure cardiac output?
(Don't forget to mention clinical aspects first, e.g. skin colour and temperature, pulse rate and volume, blood pressure, urine output, level of consciousness etc.)
What are the causes of a reduced cardiac output?
How does the body compensate for a fall in cardiac output?

(o) What is a Valsalva manoeuvre?

What would be the effects on pulse and blood pressure during a Valsalva manoeuvre?
What are the causes of an abnormal Valsalva manoeuvre?

(p) What is the Fick principle?

How would you use the Fick principle to measure renal blood flow?
What is the normal value for renal blood flow?
How are renal blood flow and glomerular filtration rate related to renal perfusion pressure?

(q) Explain how the renal tubular cell reabsorbs bicarbonate.

If you can, it might be a good idea to show this graphically, talking while you draw.

Would the urine be acidic or alkaline in the following situations:

Respiratory acidosis.
Metabolic acidosis.
Metabolic alkalosis.
Metabolic alkalosis in the presence of hypokalaemia.
Hyperkalaemia.
Hyperaldosteronism.

If you don't know the answer to these straight away, there is nothing wrong with working it out aloud so the examiner can listen to your thought process. If you happen to know the answers before you go into the exam it is still a good idea to let the examiner hear how you work it out. For one thing, it wastes time.

3. Physics, safety and clinical measurement

(a) What electrically related hazards in the operating theatre do you know about?

You should think about this before you go into the exam. It is a very common question. Divide the causes into mains related (macro and micro-shock), static related (micro-shock and explosions) and diathermy related (electrocution and burns). You could then go on to describe these in a little more detail.

What are the clinical effects of electrocution?
What factors influence the clinical effects of electrocution?
What features of the operating theatre and anaesthetic equipment reduce the risk of electric shock and the build-up of static electricity?
What factors influence the risk of explosions in the operating theatre from volatile anaesthetics?

(b) You are shown a photograph of a TEC 3 vaporizer.

What are its salient features?
What variables is it calibrated to compensate for?
How does it do this?

(c) Define saturated vapour pressure (SVP).

How does SVP vary with ambient temperature?
What is the splitting ratio?
What would be the splitting ratio to deliver 3% halothane?
At altitude where the atmospheric pressure is 0.5 atmospheres, how would you set a vaporizer to deliver enflurane to have the same anaesthetic effect as 1% enflurane at sea level?

(d) What is latent heat of vaporization?

What are the clinical reasons for humidifying inspired anaesthetic gases?
What methods are available for humidifying anaesthetic gases?
Which is most efficient and what are the hazards related to each?
What other methods are available for reducing heat loss in the unconscious patient?

(e) Describe the physical principles involved in the functioning of a Rotameter.

What factors affect its accuracy?
Why is the scale printed on the Rotameter non-linear?
What are the hazards associated with Rotameters?
How could the design of the anaesthetic machine be altered to prevent the delivery of a hypoxic mixture if the N_2O Rotameter cracks?

(f) You are shown a Wright's respirometer.

Describe it.
Draw the internal working parts.
What factors affect its accuracy?

(When you're in theatre before the exam, practise talking about all the pieces of equipment you can find. Ask your ODA to dig up old bits of equipment for you to look at and ask them what they are. ODAs are a wealth of knowledge. In the viva you may be shown various objects to describe. They are often small as they fit easily into an examiner's pocket. Examples include Touhy needles, filling keys, valves, endotracheal tubes of all types and their connectors and oxygen failure alarms. If you know what it is, tell the examiner what it is and then describe it. On the other hand, you may never have seen one before. Don't panic. Just describe what you see and make an intelligent guess as to what it may be used for.)

(g) What is the difference between a vapour and a gas?

What is critical temperature?
What is the critical temperature of nitrous oxide?
What happens to the outside of a nitrous oxide cylinder during continuous use?
Why does this occur?
Describe the changes you would see on a nitrous oxide cylinder's pressure gauge during continuous use?
How can you estimate the amount of nitrous oxide left in a cylinder?

(h) What ventilator do you use in your practice?

Don't make up a ventilator. Tell the truth.

How do you classify ventilators?
How does the (ventilator you have chosen) work?
Why does the Manley ventilator have two bellows?
What sort of ventilator is it?
What are its limitations?

(i) What methods are available for measuring the state of oxygenation of an anaesthetized patient?

Think clinical first. Don't forget the obvious like cyanosis.

How does the pulse oximeter work?
What are its advantages and disadvantages?
How would you measure the partial pressure of oxygen in plasma?
What are the features of a carbon dioxide electrode?
How does a mass spectrometer work?

(j) What are the principles of measuring expired gases and vapours during anaesthesia?

(k) What features of the anaesthetic machine protect the patient from barotrauma?

Draw the internal workings of a pressure reducing valve.

(l) What features of the supply of gases protect the patient from receiving a hypoxic mixture?

You must mention pipelines, cylinders and Rotameters. You should also mention alarms which warn of failure of oxygen supply, e.g. oxygen analysers and ventilator alarms as well as pulse oximeters which detect hypoxia.

What is a Bodok seal?
What is the pin index system?
Where are 'O' rings found and what do they do?

(m) Describe how you would check an anaesthetic machine.

The college gives guidelines about this.
Start with the oxygen analyser. How does it work? How do you zero it?

What are the pressures in the cylinders?
What are cylinders made of?
What is the tare weight of a cylinder?
What does cracking the cylinder mean?

(n) What methods are available for reducing atmospheric pollution in the operating theatre?

Remember, you can either remove gas, e.g. scavenging, or use less gas, e.g. circle systems, regional techniques.

(o) Draw a Bain circuit.

Make sure you draw it correctly and big enough.

How do you ensure that the inner tube is not disconnected?
What flows are required to prevent rebreathing in the sponta-
neously breathing and ventilated patient?
What is an Ayre's t-piece?

(p) How do you measure blood pressure?

You must know the direct and indirect ways and their limitations.

4. Clinical topics

These are often more difficult to answer well than they appear.
Don't be afraid to tell the examiner how you would actually
approach an anaesthetic and try to imagine yourself back at work
faced with the situation the examiner has set for you. So as to
organize your answer try to categorize it first.

For example, all operations can be done under general, regional
or local anaesthesia or a combination of all three.

The anaesthetic involves induction, maintenance and monitoring, reversal and postoperative care, particularly pain relief,
oxygen therapy, HDU and ITU.

The anaesthetic depends on patient factors, e.g. disease state,
age, surgical factors, e.g. blood loss, duration, position, and anaesthetic factors, e.g. difficult intubation, regional techniques.

(a) What are the problems with anaesthetizing a patient for a
TURP?

Problems with surgery:

Haemorrhage.
Hypervolaemia.
Hyponatraemia.
Haemolysis.
Hypothermia.

Problems with patient:

Age.
Concurrent disease.
Renal failure.

Problems with the anaesthetic:

GA – endotracheal tube? Ventilated or spontaneously breathing.
Regional – spinal, epidural, caudal.

(b) How would you perform an epidural?

The answer to any local block question can be divided into headings beginning with the letter 'p' (with a few others added at the end). If you answer the question like this you will score loads of marks before you even get to performing the procedure itself.

Preoperative visit and assessment including

(i) Explanation of the procedure.
(ii) Exclusion of contraindications.
(iii) Verbal or written consent.

Premedication.
Preparation of:

(i) Yourself (gown, gloves etc.).
(ii) The anaesthetic room (resus equipment, drugs for induction and intubation if required).
(iii) The patient (gain intravenous access).

Positioning of the patient and preparing the skin.
Procedure and anatomical landmarks:

(i) Needle type (gauge, length etc.).
(ii) Technique (loss of resistance to air/saline, direction of needle etc.).
(iii) Local anaesthetic (type, concentration, amount, additives etc.).
(iv) Don't forget to aspirate for blood before you inject!!

Expected effect (e.g. numbness and weakness in the legs).
Side effects (e.g. intravenous injection causing peri-oral tingling, convulsion etc.).
Recovery (including monitoring and care of catheters).

(c) You are called to casualty. A man has been stabbed in the right side of his chest with a bread knife.

How would you manage this patient?

Remember that in ALL questions about emergencies you must mention assessment of 'Airway, Breathing, Circulation' first!!!!
You are, after all, an anaesthetist.

What problems would you anticipate?
What are the signs of a tension pneumothorax?
How would you manage it?
Why cannulate the second intercostal space?
What are the signs of cardiac tamponade?
How would you manage it?
What are the signs of hypovolaemia?

(d) You are called to recovery where a patient is not breathing following a total abdominal hysterectomy under GA.

What would you do (remember 'A, B, C')?
What is the differential diagnosis?
How does a peripheral nerve stimulator work?
How would you treat this patient?

(e) You are visiting your patients preoperatively and have just seen a patient who is scheduled to have an open cholecystectomy. As you get up to leave, she asks you about pain relief after the operation. What methods are available for postoperative pain relief in this patient?

This is still a trendy topic, so you must prepare something in advance. It is advisable to categorize your answer, e.g. by routes of administration. Have something prepared about acute pain teams.

(f) A 7-year-old child who has recently had a tonsillectomy is to come back to theatre because he is bleeding from the tonsillar bed. How are you going to approach this patient?

THIS QUESTION IS ONE OF THE OLD CHESTNUTS!!!!

Others include penetrating eye injuries in a patient with a full stomach, management of a failed intubation and anaesthesia in patients with upper airway obstruction.

IF YOU CAN'T ANSWER THESE QUESTIONS CONFIDENTLY ON THE DAY OF THE EXAM YOU WILL PROBABLY FAIL!!!

So, with that in mind, prepare the answers to these chestnuts before the exam. There is nothing worse than thinking about these for the first time on the day of the exam.

Often, as in the case of the bleeding tonsil, there is more than one way to approach the problem, e.g. inhalational induction in left lateral position versus IV induction with cricoid pressure.

Choose one of these methods to describe in the exam, but be aware that there are others.

(g) What methods do you use to assess the degree of difficulty to expect in intubating a patient?

How reliable are these tests?
What patient features are associated with difficulty to intubate?

Classify before you answer, e.g. congenital, anatomical, disease processes.

How do you grade the difficulty at the time of intubation?
How would you manage a patient who you knew was a grade 4 laryngoscopy the last time they were anaesthetized by one of your consultants?

(h) While visiting your patients preoperatively, you are faced with the following patients. How would you manage them?

(i)   A non-insulin dependent diabetic for extraction of a cataract.
(ii) A patient with a blood pressure of 185/110 for repair of an inguinal hernia.
(iii) A 24-year-old girl for ERPC with a haemoglobin of 9 g/dl.
(iv) A 79-year-old asymptomatic patient for a total abdominal hysterectomy with q waves in lead II, III and aVf on the ECG.

(i) During a mastectomy in a ventilated patient, the capnograph alarms because the end expiratory carbon dioxide has fallen to zero. What are the possible causes?

Classify before you answer, e.g. respiratory or cardiac causes.

How would you diagnose the cause?
What would you do?
What are the signs of an air embolus?
How would you manage an air embolus in this patient?

N.B. This question could be about any intraoperative emergency, e.g. asystole, anaphylaxis, hypotension, hypoxia, disconnection etc. You must be able to tell the examiner what you would do almost without thinking. The examiner may try to put pressure on you to make things more realistic (it's all part of the game). So, it is vital that you think about these situations before the exam.

(j) What are the problems associated with anaesthetizing a patient with rheumatoid arthritis?

(k) Have you anaesthetized a patient in the prone position? What problems did you have to overcome?

(l) You have to anaesthetize a patient for a thyroidectomy. Describe your anaesthetic management?

How would you assess this patient preoperatively?
What investigations would you order?
How would you induce anaesthesia in this patient?
What sort of endotracheal tube would you use and why?
How would you maintain anaesthesia in this patient?
How would you manage emergence and extubation?
What are the possible complications associated with this procedure?

(m) How do you assess blood loss during major operations?

What are the clinical signs of hypovolaemia?
How would you manage a hypovolaemic patient during a general anaesthetic?
What are the complications of blood transfusion?

(n) What are the causes of DVT?

What methods are available to reduce the risk?
What are the signs of pulmonary embolism occurring per-operatively?
How would you manage a patient who has a massive pulmonary embolus peroperatively?

In conclusion, remember to 'talk the specialty' as much as you can before the exam. The nature of anaesthesia can make you non-communicative, but you must practice discussing the subject when-ever you can.

5

The objectively structured clinical examination (OSCE)

OSCE stands for Objective Structured Clinical Examination. It was not part of the old part one exam. Therefore, at the time of writing this book, the OSCE is new to you and to us. Having said that, the College Tutors have had the nature of the OSCEs clearly explained to them, so do not hesitate to ask them. We shall outline the OSCE syllabus and present the principles involved in coping with this part of the exam. We shall also present examples of the situations that will appear in the real exam.

The OSCE is objective. This means that at the stations where the examiner is present, he is there merely as an observer. He is to be treated as simply a fly on the wall. He will have a checklist to fill in to assess whether you are dealing with the station adequately. For example, if you are asked to perform an epidural on a model, you will be expected to perform the block as if it were your everyday practice. The examiner will check that you explain the procedure to the model, position the model correctly, clean the skin etc. He should not ask you any questions and you should direct yourself to the model and not to the examiner. So don't tell the examiner that 'I would explain the procedure to the patient . . .', instead tell the model 'I am going to perform an epidural on you and this will involve . . .'.

The OSCE is structured. This means that all the candidates should be faced with the same problems.

Some stations will be manned by an examiner and others will not. At each station you will be given brief instructions as to what is expected of you. All you need to do to pass is to carry these instructions out.

Assessment will take place over 2 h. There will be 16 OSCE stations. That's about 7 min in each station. You will have 30 s to get to the station, 1½ min to either read about or have the OSCE station explained to you. You will then have 5 min to complete the OSCE itself. So you don't have much time.

The stations will test you on the following topics:

Resuscitation.
Anatomy.
Regional block.
Examination.
Communication.
Data interpretation.
Equipment.
Monitoring.
Hazards.

Often these topics will be combined at one station, e.g. anatomy/ local blocks and communication/history. There will not necessarily be an equal number of questions from each category. There may well be more from the anatomy and resuscitation category for example.

The OSCE skills directory or syllabus has been stated by the College. They have divided it up into four sections:

1. Clinical assessment.
2. Data interpretation.
3. Communication.
4. Technical skills.

1. Clinical assessment

History

- Can you take a relevant history from a patient? How does it influence your management of the anaesthetic?
- Medication – past, present, drug reactions, drug interactions, smoking, alcohol, 'recreational' drugs.
- Allergies.
- Anaesthetic history – personal, familial, airway problems, intubation difficulties.
- History of presenting complaint.
- Systematic review – respiratory, cardiovascular, musculoskeletal, gastrointestinal, renal, hepatic, endocrine, obstetric, skin, blood (haemoglobinopathies, coagulopathies).
- Congenital disorders, hereditary disorders.
- Relevant neurological history.
- Mental state.
- Pain assessment.

Physical examination

Can you examine a patient relatively quickly, looking for relevant examination abnormalities that may influence the anaesthetic?

- General state – obesity, cachexia, dehydration, anaemia, jaundice.
- Respiratory system including pleural drain sites.
- Trachea – thyroid, cricoid pressure, tracheostomy anatomy.
- Airway assessment – IMPORTANT.
- Cardiovascular system.
- Neurological signs, including charts, scores.
- Abdomen.
- Musculoskeletal.
- Vascular access – suitability of sites.
- Epidurals, spinals, caudals.
- Local nerve blocks – brachial plexus, femoral and dorsal nerve of penis.

2. Data interpretation

Can you interpret and explain the results of investigations that you look at every day?

Clinical

- Respiratory function tests.
- Exercise tolerance.
- Electrocardiographs.
- Charts including fluid balance.
- Central venous pressure.

Radiological

- Chest radiographs.
- Neck, thoracic inlet.
- Abdominal films.
- Skull films.
- Simple imaging investigations.

Laboratory tests

- Haematology, coagulation, electrophoresis.

- Electrolytes, urea.
- Renal function.
- pH and blood gases.
- Thyroid, liver, adrenal function.

3. Communication

- Are you able to clearly discuss and explain with patients the worrying aspects, and colleagues the relevant aspects of anaesthetic care?
- Consent for general and regional anaesthesia.
- Explanation of the need for preoperative screening – hepatitis, HIV, sickle cell.
- Analgesic techniques – including side effects and complications.
- Premedication.
- Postoperative explanation and care.
- Nursing orders – preoperative, premedication, postoperative care and analgesia.
- Checking of patients in theatre.
- Recovery area management, including discharge.
- Explanation to patients and relatives about:
      suxamethonium apnoea
      difficult intubation
      anaphylaxis
      malignant hyperthermia
      post-spinal headache

4. Technical skills

Clinical

- Resuscitation – ALL ASPECTS OF CARE AND MANAGEMENT.
- Venous access – CVP monitoring.
- Arterial pressure monitoring.
- Pleural drain insertion.
- Lumbar puncture/spinal anaesthesia.
- Epidural management.
- Caudals.
- Nerve blocks.
- Intravenous regional analgesia.

Equipment

Can you check, set up, and understand the common pieces of equipment that you use? If pieces are missing or wrongly connected you must be able to find out what is wrong.

- CHECKING ANAESTHETIC MACHINE.
- BREATHING SYSTEMS AND CHECKS.
- Ventilators.
- Monitoring equipment.
- Checking resuscitation equipment.
- Anaesthetic hazards.
- Equipment check lists:
  resuscitation equipment
  epidural/spinal packs
  paediatric intubation
  difficult and failed intubation kits
  failed intubation management
  arterial pressure monitoring
- Defibrillators.
- Recovery room equipment.

This completes the OSCE skills directory. It's only what you do every day except in the exam you must do it properly!!!

Examples of OSCE stations

Resuscitation

(a) There is an examiner present and you are told that this mannequin has collapsed at an Arsenal football match. You exclude boredom!! You will be asked to assess and manage this situation.

He will OBSERVE your assessment and management of cardiac arrest.

This is basic CPR, i.e. ABC, ask for help, start cardiac massage and do it according to the resuscitation council guidelines.

You will either be asked to perform this exercise on a mannequin or write down what you would do on a card. REMEMBER YOU ARE ROLE PLAYING AND SHOULD DO IN THE EXAM WHAT YOU WOULD DO IN REAL LIFE.

(b) You enter a room where there is a mannequin attached to an ECG machine which shows sinus rhythm. You are told there is no cardiac output. You are told this is electro-mechanical disassociation. You are given a card with the following questions.

(i)   Several possible causes for this need to be considered and excluded and need to be treated appropriately. Write down five of these causes.

(ii)   What is the dose of adrenaline you will need in this situation?

(iii) How many compression/ventilation sequences do you give?

(iv)   What pressor agents should you consider?

(v)   What dose of adrenaline should now be considered?

Answers

(i)   Pneumothorax, hypovolaemia, cardiac tamponade, pulmonary embolus, drug overdose, hypothermia, and electrolyte imbalance.

(ii)   1 mg.

(iii) 10.

(iv)   Calcium, bicarbonate and adrenaline.

(v)   5 mg.

(c) A mannequin is attached to an ECG which shows ventricular fibrillation. The following questions will be presented regarding the advanced management of this condition.

(i)   Do you give a precordial thump?

(ii)   The amount of joules given for initial defibrillation is . . . .?

(iii) The second defibrillation requires . . . . joules.

(iv)   The third defibrillation requires . . . . joules.

(v)   What dose of which drug is now given?

(vi)   How many compression/ventilation sequences are now given?

(vii) How many further defibrillations should be given?

(viii) How many joules should be applied?

(ix)   Adrenaline/defibrillation cycles now occur. After how many cycles do you consider further drug treatment?

(x)   What four drugs would you now consider giving?

Answers

(i)   Yes.

(ii)   200 J.

(iii) 200 J.

(iv)   360 J.

(v)   Adrenaline 1 mg.

(vi)   10.

(vii) 3.

(viii) 360 J.

(ix) 3.
(x)   Sodium bicarbonate, amiodarone, bretylium, lignocaine.

History and communication

(a) On the door of this station you will read the following clinical scenario: this patient is going to have an inguinal hernia repair on a day stay basis under general anaesthetic. You are visiting the patient preoperatively to assess him.

On entering the room you may meet an actor or the examiner who is playing the patient role. During your assessment the actor will guide you towards the object of the station. He may ask about the management of his postoperative pain or alternatively about your views on premedication. You will be examined on your explanation and your communication skills.

(b) The setting of this station is that you are asked to assess the patient's airway for intubation.

When you enter the room you may meet an actor. You will be expected to take a history and examine the patient as you would on the ward. Remember to be polite, ask about previous operations, and assess jaw opening, thyro-mental distance, dental problems, Mallampati score, Wilson risk factors and mobility of the cervical spine.

The examiner will assess the way in which you approach both the patient and the problem.

(c) You enter a room and are told the following history: A 32-year-old woman has had a manual removal of placenta under spinal anaesthesia. She is now complaining of a severe headache. An actress will play the part of the patient. Take a history from the patient and explain the causes and management of the headache to the patient.

Remember you are role playing. In the communication stations, the actor or the examiner who is playing the part of the patient will offer some information. However, you will be expected to elicit further information such as the type of headache, whether it is postural, what relieves it and what brings it on. You must clearly describe to the patient what you propose to do to manage this condition and tell the patient what the likely course of the headache will be. You will be marked by the examiner, who will be a fly on the wall, as to how you approach the patient and whether you elicit all the information you need to make a diagnosis.

(d) The scenario is a 28-year-old female patient with abdominal pain who is to have a laparoscopy for a possible torsion of an ovarian cyst as an emergency. You must take a history from her to assess her suitability for anaesthesia and discuss any problems that may arise during your questioning.

Start to take a history as you would on the ward in your hospital. The patient has been told to offer some information to you. In this case she will tell you of a problem her brother had with a minor anaesthetic after which he failed to breathe properly. A few weeks later some blood was taken from her and other relatives to look for something in the blood.

The examiner will mark you on whether you diagnose the problem (in this case suxamethonium apnoea) through your questioning, on how you explain it to the patient and on what you decide to do next.

You should find out if the patient has had any other operations and where they were, for example. You could discuss the problem with the surgeons to see if you have time to find out a little more about the enzymatic status of the patient.

Anatomy and local blocks

(a) This is a diagram of a lumbar vertebra (Figure 5.1).

(i)   Label the drawing of this lumbar vertebra.
(ii) List three contraindications to performing a lumbar epidural.
(iii) List five side effects of injecting local anaesthetic into the epidural space.
(iv) List four complications of injecting an opioid into the epidural space.

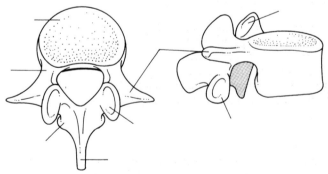

Figure 5.1 (Reproduced from Yentis, Hirsch and Smith (1995) *Anaesthesia A–Z* by permission)

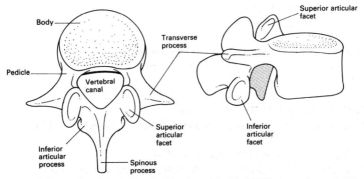

Figure 5.2 (Reproduced from Yentis, Hirsch and Smith (1995) *Anaesthesia A–Z* by permission)

Answers
(i)   See diagram (Figure 5.2).
(ii) Local sepsis, anticoagulation, patient refusal.
(iii) Hypotension, total spinal, anaphylaxis, nerve damage due to intra-neural injection, shivering.
(iv) Respiratory depression, urinary retention, itching, nausea and vomiting.

(b) This is a diagram of the larynx (Figure 5.3).

(i)   Label this diagram of the larynx.
(ii) List four indications for performing a tracheostomy.
(iii) List four early complications associated with tracheostomies.
(iv) List three late complications associated with tracheostomies.

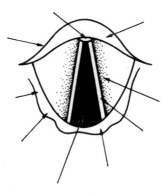

Figure 5.3 (Reproduced from Yentis, Hirsch and Smith (1995) *Anaesthesia A–Z* by permission)

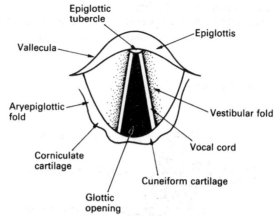

Figure 5.4 (Reproduced from Yentis, Hirsch and Smith (1995) *Anaesthesia A–Z* by permission)

Answers

(i) See diagram (Figure 5.4).

(ii) Relief of airway obstruction, to protect the lower airways from aspiration if laryngeal reflexes are absent, to allow suction, IPPV lasting longer than 3–4 weeks.

(iii) Haemorrhage, blockage of the tube, misplacement of the tube, pneumothorax.

(iv) Infection, tracheal erosion, tracheal stenosis, tracheal dilatation.

(c) This is a diagram of the brachial plexus (Figure 5.5).

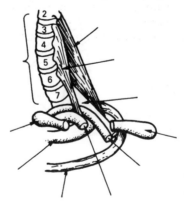

Figure 5.5 (Reproduced from Yentis, Hirsch and Smith (1995) *Anaesthesia A–Z* by permission)

(i)   Label this diagram of the brachial plexus.
(ii) List three approaches to perform a brachial plexus block.
(iii) List five complications particular to brachial plexus block.

Answers
(i)   See diagram (Figure 5.6).

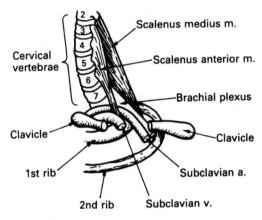

Figure 5.6 (Reproduced from Yentis, Hirsch and Smith (1995) *Anaesthesia A–Z* by permission)

(ii) Interscaline, supraclavicular, axillary.
(iii) Phrenic nerve block, recurrent laryngeal nerve block, Horner's syndrome, inadvertent spinal or epidural block, injection into the vertebral artery, injection into the subclavian artery, pneumothorax, and injection into the axillary artery.

Data interpretation

(a) This 70-kg patient has been brought to casualty in a semi-concious state. You have no further information other than these blood gases:

pH 7.21
PO_2 10.3 kPa
PCO_2 2.7 kPa
HCO_3 19 mmol/l
BE −8

(i)   What type of acidosis is shown by these blood gases?
(ii) List five possible causes that would produce these blood gases?
(iii) What is the initial compensation mechanism for the acidosis illustrated by these blood gases?
(iv) Would you give this patient sodium bicarbonate?
(v)   If the pH fell to 7.06 and the base excess fell to −15, how many mmols of sodium bicarbonate would you recommend?

Answers
(i)   Metabolic acidosis.
(ii) Ketoacidosis due to diabetes.
      Lactic acidosis due to shock.
      Acid ingestion (aspirin poisoning).
      Reduced acid excretion in acute renal failure.
      Increased bicarbonate loss, e.g. diarrhoea, ureteroenterostomy.
(iii) Hyperventilation.
(iv) No. (Generally people don't give sodium bicarbonate until the pH falls below 7.1.)
(v)   350 mmol. This is 350 ml of 8.4% sodium bicarbonate. To work this out use the following equation:

mmol of bicarbonate required = Base excess × body weight (kg) ÷ 3

In this case $15 \times 70 \div 3 = 350$ mmol.

(b) You are shown the following set of clotting study results from a patient scheduled for elective total hip replacement:

Platelets	$350 \times 10^9/l$
PT	35 s
PTTK (APTT)	95 s
TT	11 s

(i)   What are the normal values for these tests?
(ii) Which of these test the extrinsic coagulation pathway?
(iii) Which of these test the intrinsic coagulation pathway?
(iv) Which of these test the common coagulation pathway?
(v)   Which part of the coagulation pathway does thrombin time (TT) test?
(vi) Which anticoagulant is this patient likely to be taking?
(vii) How should this patient be managed preoperatively regarding his coagulation status?

Answers
(i) Platelets: $150–400 \times 10^9/l$.
     PT: 11–15 s.
     PTTK: 35–40 s.
     TT: 10–15 s.
(ii) PT.
(iii) PTTK.
(iv) PT and PTTK.
(v) Conversion of fibrinogen to fibrin.
(vi) Warfarin (heparin increase TT as well).
(vii) Discontinue warfarin therapy (with heparin cover if required). Give vitamin K or fresh frozen plasma.

(c) You are shown this diagram (Figure 5.7) of four ECG traces which you may see in a patient under general anaesthesia. The upper trace (a) is normal.

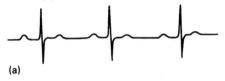

(a)

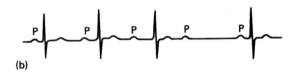

(b)

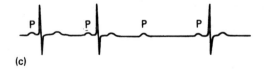

(c)

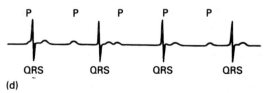

(d)

Figure 5.7 (Reproduced from Yentis, Hirsch and Smith (1995) *Anaesthesia A–Z* by permission)

(i)   What is the abnormality in traces (b) to (d)?
(ii) What is the ECG definition of first degree heart block?
(iii) List five causes of heart block in the anaesthetized patient?
(iv) What is the drug of choice in the treatment of third degree heart block?
(v)   What is the dose of this drug?
(vi) What is the next line of management for the treatment of third degree heart block?

Answers
(i)   b: 2nd degree heart block (Mobitz I or Wenckebach phenomenon).
      c: 2nd degree heart block (Mobitz II).
      d: 3rd degree heart block.
(ii) P-R interval greater than 0.2 s.
(iii) Ageing, ischaemic heart disease, increased vagal tone, halothane, digoxin, cardiomyopathy, myocarditis, beta blockers, hyperkalaemia, and congenital heart block.
(iv) Isoprenaline.
(v)   0.02–0.2 (μg/kg/min).
(vi) Electrical cardiac pacing.

Equipment and monitoring

(a) Look at this diagram of breathing circuits (Figure 5.8).

(i)   Using the letters A–F, label this diagram of breathing circuits according to the Mapleson classification of breathing systems.
(ii) Which system is most efficient for spontaneous ventilation in adults?
(iii) How is the co-axial version of the Mapleson A otherwise known?
(iv) Which of these systems is most commonly used in the transfer of ventilated patients and resuscitation?
(v)   In ml/kg per min, what fresh gas flow rates will prevent rebreathing in a spontaneously breathing 70-kg patient using a Mapleson A breathing system?
(vi) In terms of minute ventilation, what fresh gas flows are required to prevent rebreathing in spontaneously breathing patients using the Mapleson D breathing system?
(vii) Which breathing system is also called the Jackson Rees modification?

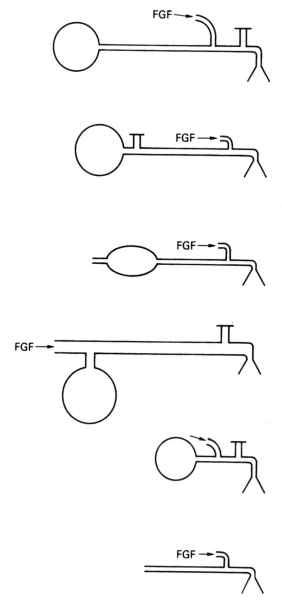

Figure 5.8 (Reproduced from Yentis, Hirsch and Smith (1995) *Anaesthesia A–Z* by permission)

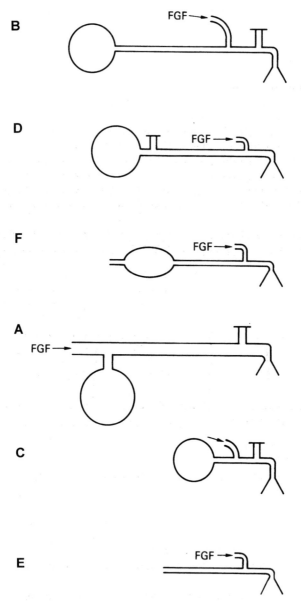

Figure 5.9 (Reproduced from Yentis, Hirsch and Smith (1995) *Anaesthesia A–Z* by permission)

Answers
(i)   See the diagram (Figure 5.9).
(ii)   A.
(iii) Lack.
(iv)   C.
(v)   70.
(vi)   2–3 × minute volume.
(vii) F.

(b) You enter a station where there is an anaesthetic machine. The examiner asks you to check the machine.

You must be able to do this according to the College guidelines without even thinking about it.

There may well be something wrong with the machine, e.g. missing 'O' ring from the vaporizer, missing Bodok seal.

(c) This diagram shows the normal trace of end-tidal CO_2 seen on a capnograph in a ventilated anaesthetized patient (Figure 5.10).

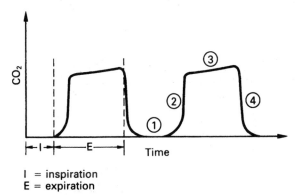

I = inspiration
E = expiration

Figure 5.10 (Reproduced from Yentis, Hirsch and Smith (1995) *Anaesthesia A–Z* by permission)

(i)   Label 1–4.
(ii)   What may cause a raised baseline?
(iii) What causes excessive sloping of the upstroke (phase 2 in the diagram)?
(iv)   What would cause the plateau (phase 3 in the diagram) to slope upwards?
(v)   List 5 causes for the end-tidal CO_2 to fall to zero.

Answers
(i)   1 = zero baseline during inspiration.
       2 = appearance of alveolar gas.
       3 = mixing of alveolar gas.
       4 = onset of inspiration.
(ii)   Rebreathing.
(iii) Obstruction to expiration, e.g. asthma.
(iv)   Unequal mixing of alveolar gas, e.g. COAD.
(v)   Pulmonary embolus.
       Air embolus.
       Cardiac arrest.
       Disconnection of breathing system.
       Obstruction of breathing system.

Hazards

(a) You are anaesthetizing an ASA 1 adult patient for a total abdominal hysterectomy. The patient is ventilated. After 30 min the airway pressure in this patient rises to 45 cm H_2O.

(i)   List five causes for the sudden rise in airway pressure in this patient.
(ii)   What is the dose of salbutamol you would give if you suspected bronchospasm?
(iii) What is the bolus dose of aminophylline you would then give if bronchospasm failed to settle?
(iv)   Following the bolus of aminophylline, what infusion rate would you commence?

Answers
(i)   Blocked end-tracheal tube (ETT).
       Herniation of ETT cuff.
       Kinked ETT.
       Kinked tubing from ventilator.
       Insufficient neuromuscular paralysis.
       Light anaesthesia.
       Pulmonary oedema.
       Pneumothorax.
       Bronchospasm.
       Malignant hyperpyrexia.
(ii)   250 μg.
(iii) 3–6 mg/kg.
(iv)   0.5 mg/kg per h.

(b) You are shown a picture of a diathermy machine.

(i)   What is the frequency of the electrical current used in surgical diathermy?
(ii) What is unipolar diathermy?
(iii) What is bipolar diathermy?
(iv) List four complications associated with the use of diathermy.
(v)   How may the risk of patient electrocution be reduced?

Answers
(i)   0.5–1 MHz.
(ii) Forceps etc. act as one electrode and the patient plate acts as another.
(iii) Current passes through tissue from one limb of the forceps to the other (no patient plate is required).
(iv) Patient burn due to incorrect placement of patient plate.
      Patient burn due to activation of the forceps while they are touching another part of the patient or lying in a pool of blood or saline on the patient.
      Electrocution of the patient. If the patient plate is earthed, current may take another route to earth, e.g. through a metal drip stand, which the patient may be touching, leading to electrocution.
      Ignition spark for combustible anaesthetic vapours and gases.
      Pacemaker interference.
(v)   Isolate the diathermy from earth so that stray current can no longer flow through the patient to earth.

(c) You are shown the following blood gas results from an ASA I patient undergoing internal fixation of a fractured ankle breathing spontaneously under general anaesthesia.

pH	7.23
pCO_2	9 kPa
pO_2	15 kPa
Bicarbonate	27 mmol/l
BE	+2

(i)   What is the most striking abnormality?
(ii) List five causes for the abnormality.
(iii) List five clinical signs that may be present.

Answers

(i)   raised pCO_2.

(ii)   Opiates causing hypoventilation.
       Anaesthetic volatile agents causing hypoventilation.
       Rebreathing CO_2 through breathing circuit.
       V/Q mismatch, e.g. COAD.
       Malignant hyperpyrexia.
       Release of hydrogen ions following deflation of tourniquet.
       Sepsis causing acidosis.

(iii) Increased respiratory rate.
       Increased tidal volume.
       Tachycardia.
       Hypertension.
       Arrhythmias.
       Sweating.
       Dilated pupils.

In conclusion, the OSCEs test your knowledge and clinical
acumen. They eliminate examiner bias and test your practical and
theoretical skills and your ability to communicate with patients
and colleagues.

Reference

Yentis, S. M., Hirsch, N. P. and Smith, G. B. (1995) *Anaesthesia A–Z*, Butterworth-
Heinemann, Oxford.

Index

Anaesthesia A–Z
An Encyclopaedia of Principles and Practice

S Yentis BSc MD BS FRCA
Consultant Anaesthetist, Chelsea and Westminster Hospital,
London, UK

N Hirsch MB BS FRCA
Consultant Anaesthetist and Honorary Senior Lecturer, The
National Hospital for Neurology and Neurosurgery, Queen
Street, London, UK

G Smith BM FRCA
Consultant Anaesthetist and Director of Intensive Care Services,
Queen Alexandra Hospital, Portsmouth, UK

An encyclopaedic source of information on all aspects of
anaesthesia and pain control in a concise, alphabetical format.

'. . . a huge amount of easily accessible and readable factual
information on all aspects of anaesthesia in a single volume.'
Anaesthesia

'The information presented is up-to-date, practical and clinically
relevant . . . anaesthetists in general and examination candidates
in particular may find [it] valuable as a spot check for current
knowledge'. *British Medical Journal*

'I can recommend this book to all libraries and to those
candidates who want to be able to converse on equal terms with
even the most perverse of examiners'. *British Journal of
Anaesthesia*

1995 480pp 270 × 202mm 150 line illustrations
PAPERBACK 0 7506 2285 7 £35.00

Basic Physics and Measurement in Anaesthesia
Fourth Edition

G D Parbrook MD RRARCS
Formerly Senior Lecturer, University of Glasgow, Department of
Anaesthesia, The Royal Infirmary, Glasgow, UK

P D Davis BSc CPhys MIstP MIPSM
Principal Physicist, West Scotland Health Boards' Department of
Clinical Physics and Bio-Engineering, Glasgow, UK

G Kenny BSc MD FRCA
Senior Lecturer, Department of Anaesthesia, University of
Glasgow, Head of Anaesthesia, HCI International, Glasgow

New for the Fourth Edition

* Comprehensively revised and updated
* New section on magnetic resonance imaging
* Additional material on monitoring depth of anaesthesia
* Descriptions of new apparatus, with the retention of
  information on older types of equipment where important for
  the demonstration of physical principles

Previous edition review from *Anaesthesia and Intensive Care*:
' . . . an eminently readable source of information on the physics
of anaesthesia and its associated measurements'.

1995 380pp 234 × 156mm Illustrated
PAPERBACK 0 7506 1713 6 £32.50

Understanding Anaesthesia
Third Edition

Len E S Carrie MB ChB FRCA DA
Consultant Anaesthetist, Nuffield Department of Anaesthetics,
Oxford Radcliffe Hospitals and Clinical Lecturer, University of
Oxford, UK

Peter J Simpson MBBS MD MRCS LRCP FRCA
Consultant Anaesthetist, Frenchay Hospital, Bristol and Senior
Clinical Lecturer, Department of Anaesthesia, University of
Bristol, UK

Mansukh T Popat MB BS FRCA
Consultant Anaesthetist, Nuffield Department of Anaesthetics,
Oxford Radcliffe Hospitals, Oxford, UK

'Medical students and new entrants to anaesthesia will find this
book gives an excellent flavour of what the speciality is about. I
highly recommend it.' *British Journal of Hospital Medicine*

1996 432pp 234 × 156mm Illustrated
PAPERBACK 0 7506 2079 X £25.00

Lee's Synopsis of Anaesthesia
Eleventh Edition

R S Atkinson OBE MA MB BChir FRCAnaes
Honorary Consulting Anaesthetist, Southend Hospital, Southend,
UK

G B Rushman MB BS FRCAnaes
Consultant Anaesthetist, Southend Hospital, Southend, UK

N J H Davies MA DM MRCP FRCA
Consultant Anaesthetist, Southampton General Hospital,
Southampton, UK

An encyclopaedic reference text for the clinical anaesthetist,
incorporating all that is relevant within the speciality in a
structured, concise and instructive way.

'THE favourite British anaesthetic text, matured rather than
aged, packed with information, the only book to buy. The
eleventh edition is no exception to the previous high standard,
you should buy one . . .' *Today's Anaesthetist*

1993 912pp 234 × 156mm Illustrated
HARDBACK 0 7506 1449 8 £40.00